Instructor's Manual

Geronto _____y
Nursing

FIFTH EDITION

Charlotte Eliopoulos, RNC, MPH, PhD
Specialist in Holistic Gerontological Care
President, Health Education Network
Glen Arm, Maryland

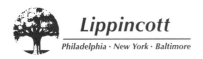

Lippincott
Philadelphia · New York · Baltimore

Ancillary Editor	Doris S. Wray
Compositor:	LWW
Printer/Binder:	R.R. Donnelley

Fifth Edition

ISBN: 0-7817-2819-3

Preface

The fifth edition of *Gerontological Nursing* by Charlotte Eliopoulos is accompanied by a new instructor's manual designed to assist instructors in leading students through a meaningful learning experience in an efficient, creative manner. This manual provides faculty with the essence of the material presented in each chapter and guidance in helping students understand a dynamic, holistic nursing role with elders.

The 38 chapters of *Gerontological Nursing* are divided into four units. Units I and II focus on issues pertaining to health aging and wellness promotion of elders. Common geriatric conditions and the concerns they create for nurses are addressed in Units III and IV. This new edition highlights holistic nursing principles and practices that assist students in integrating the art and science of caring and healing with conventional treatments of health conditions. While gaining appreciation of medical and surgical interventions what can enhance the quality and quantity of elders' lives in profound ways, students also will be encouraged to recognize the unique healing role that nurses can develop in gerontological care. Because those who serve as healers to others must be attentive to their own health and healing, a new feature, *Points to Ponder,* which challenges students to explore the meaning of the theory to their own lives has been added to the text. Instructors should encourage students to invest time in thoughtful consideration of these points and discuss their responses.

ORGANIZATION OF INSTRUCTOR'S MANUAL

The manual consists of 38 chapters, each corresponding to a chapter in the text. Each chapter includes:

- **Chapter Overview:** A summary of the content covered in the chapter.
- **Significant Displays, Tables, and Figures:** A list of tabular, boxed, or displayed material for each chapter listed for easy reference.
- **Student Objectives:** A listing of outcomes that the students should experience from the chapter.
- **Classroom Teaching-Learning Activities:** Discussion questions, classroom activities, and written assignments.
- **Guidelines for Evaluating Critical Thinking Exercises:** A discussions of possible responses that students could offer to the Critical Thinking Exercises at the end of each chapter.
- **Test Questions:** Ten questions are provided for each chapter.

It is recognized that gerontological nursing material is taught in a variety of ways, ranging from a several-day elective to integrated content within other courses to a full-semester course. For this reason, learning needs and teaching strategies will vary. A variety of teaching ideas are offered to meet the diverse needs of different groups. However, the theory within the text becomes most meaningful and lasting when made to "come alive" by an instructor who demonstrates enthusiasm, commitment, and sensitivity to the significance of holistic nursing of older adults.

Peace and Blessings
Charlotte Eliopoulos

Contents

UNIT III
Common Geriatric Conditions

UNIT IV
Gerontological Care Issues

Foundations of Nursing an Aging Population

This section presents basic facts to offer a foundation to understanding gerontological nursing. Chapter 1, Framework for Gerontological Nursing, gives a historical perspective of the development of views about the aged and their care. It then proceeds to discuss the standards and principles upon which gerontological nursing practice is built and the major roles that can be assumed by nurses in this specialty. The concept of holistic gerontological nursing care, introduced in this chapter, is a new feature in this edition that is woven throughout the entire text.

Information presented in Chapter 2, Facts About the Aging Population, aids the reader in separating myths from realities about the elderly. Characteristics of today's aged population and projections for tomorrow's elderly population are reviewed.

Popular biological and psychosocial theories of aging are presented in Chapter 3, Theories of Aging, in an effort to not only aid students in understanding the theories but also assist them to identify factors that positively and negatively affect the aging process.

Chapter 4, Cultural Diversity, surveys the unique views of major ethnic groups toward the aged, health, and healing. The general theme is that nurses need to appreciate the diversity found among older adults and accommodate care accordingly rather than expect the elderly to conform to a single profile.

Life changes and the related effect on lifestyle are reviewed in Chapter 5, Life Transitions. The shift in roles and responsibilities between parents and children and the challenges faced by widows are the major family changes discussed. The impact of retirement on status, role, identity, and income is considered. Students are encouraged to see a role for nursing intervention as part of health promotion in each phase of retirement. Students are provided with life review and reminiscence as strategies to assist older adults as the awareness of mortality becomes increasingly acute. The impact of the reality of declining function one faces with age is presented, with general suggestions for nursing intervention. (Future chapters will review in-depth nursing interventions for specific age-related changes and health problems.) Nursing considerations to assist elders in dealing with reduced income, their shrinking social world, and societal prejudice are included.

Common Aging Changes, Chapter 6, states major changes to each body system and common psychological changes. Because later chapters will provide detailed descriptions of nursing actions that assist elders in compensating for age-related changes and that promote health, the discussion in this chapter is limited to the changes experienced by the older adult.

This unit should assist the student in gaining an appreciation of the opportunities and challenges related to nursing aging adults—an appreciation that can serve as the foundation for gerontological nursing practice.

Framework for Gerontological Nursing

Chapter 1 presents an introduction to the care of the aged and to nursing's relationship to this arena. A historical overview illustrates the evolution of thought concerning views toward elder members of society. The early involvement of nurses in the care of the aged is discussed to reflect nursing's interest and commitment to this group long before gerontology and geriatrics became areas of popular interest within other disciplines.

In discussing the growth of the specialty of gerontological nursing, the issue of the stigma attached to gerontological nurses in the past is honestly discussed to enable students to appreciate the past that needed to be overcome and nurses' responsibility in influencing the status of a specialty. Facts pertaining to the proliferation of literature, the development of standards, and the movement toward subspecialization of gerontological nursing are presented to reinforce the relative "youngness" of the specialty and the potential for nurses to influence its development as gerontological nursing continues to evolve.

Roles in which nurses function with older adults are reviewed. In addition to the roles of caregiver, educator, advocate, and innovator that have been included in earlier editions, this edition of *Gerontological Nursing* highlights the role of healer. This theme is set in Chapter 1 and follows in subsequent chapters, promoting nursing's historical emphasis on nurturance, comfort, empathy, and intuition as having a legitimate place in contemporary gerontological nursing.

The reader is introduced to the American Nurses Association Standards of Gerontological Nursing Practice, which are unique in that they are developed solely by and for nurses. Likewise, principles guiding the specialty are discussed.

The tapestry of holistic gerontological nursing care that will be woven throughout the book begins in this chapter. The importance of attending to the needs of the whole person—mind, body, and spirit—rather than focusing merely on the treatment of disease is emphasized.

■ Significant Displays, Tables, and Figures

Publicly Supported Programs of Benefit to Older Americans (Table 1-1)
Landmarks in the Growth of Gerontological Nursing (Table 1-2)
Gerontological Nursing Roles (Display 1-1)
Standards of Gerontological Nursing Practice (Display 1-2)

Principles of Gerontological Nursing Practice (Display 1-3)
Information System of the Gerontological Nurse (Figure 1-1)

STUDENT OBJECTIVES

After reading this chapter, the student should be able to:

1. Describe the different ways in which the aged were viewed throughout history.
2. List landmarks that affected the development of gerontological nursing.
3. Discuss major roles in gerontological nursing.
4. Identify standards utilized in gerontological nursing practice.
5. List principles guiding gerontological nursing practice.
6. Explain holistic gerontological nursing care.

■ Classroom Teaching-Learning Activities

1. Ask students to identify and discuss various ways in which the aged have been portrayed in art and literature over time.
2. Discuss factors internal and external to nursing that influenced the stigma associated with gerontological nursing in the past.
3. Discuss examples of each of the roles in which gerontological nursing can function.
4. Review consumers' recent interest in alternative and holistic health practices and challenges presented by this to gerontological nursing practice.

■ Guidelines for Evaluating Critical Thinking Exercises

1.

- higher standard of living enjoyed by society in general
- improved economic conditions
- greater knowledge and understanding of aging
- increased power base and political clout of elders
- heightened concern for all minorities and special groups

2.
- gerontological nursing not a recognized specialty
- low status of elderly in society; ageism
- poor working conditions and salaries in geriatric care settings
- poor reputation of nursing homes in the past

3.
- Most problems of elders are chronic in nature. It is less the medical management than the coming to terms with living effectively and in harmony with chronic conditions that is the challenge.
- It is important for elders to explore the spiritual and psychological aspects of their lives (e.g., developing sense of integrity, finding meaning and purpose).

4. The older adult takes an active role in all aspects of care.

5.
- crosses many specialties (psychiatry, GYN, medical-surgical)
- most needs of elders fall within realm of nursing to independent address

6.
- integration and harmony of body, mind, and spirit
- interaction of all parts of self
- interaction of self with others and universe as a whole

■ Test Questions

1. Which is a true statement regarding public support of programs to benefit the aged?
   a. Despite the proposal in 1900 for pension laws to protect the elderly, to date no state has enacted such a law.
   b. **The 1935 Social Security Act included the Federal Old Age Insurance Law.**
   c. Medicare for the aged was enacted in 1935 as the major thrust of the Social Security Act.
   d. The 1965 Older Americans' Act launched the foundation for the first White House Conference on Aging.

2. The healer role of the nurse:
   a. is based on the philosophy that nurses heal others through prayer
   b. was developed in recent years with the growth of holistic nursing

    c. views the physician as having an insignificant role in health care

    d. was apparent in early nursing practice

3. All of the following represent principles of gerontological nursing practice except:

    a. Universal self-care demands of the aged are different from other age groups

    b. Aging is a natural process common to all living organisms

    c. A variety of factors influence the aging process

    d. Unique knowledge and data are used in applying the nursing process to the older population

4. Historically, views toward the aged could be described as:

    a. positive in being laced with an attitude of respect for elders

    b. running the gamut from positive to negative

    c. negative in viewing old age as a dreaded disease

    d. unknown due to the relatively small proportion of elders

5. The decade of the 20th century that saw gerontological nursing become a recognized specialty through the American Nurses Association was the:

    a. 1930s

    b. 1960s

    c. 1970s

    d. 1990s

6. *Standards of Gerontological Nursing Practice* was first published in:

    a. 1950

    b. 1960

    c. 1970

    d. 1980

7. Inherent in the implementation of gerontological nursing practice are the standards regarding the:

    a. active participation of older adults and their significant others

    b. professional's responsibility to make good decisions for the older adult

    c. importance of nursing assuming a role above all other disciplines

    d. need to prepare older adults for inevitable disability and decline

8. Responsibility for the gerontological nurse's professional development rests with:
   a. the general nursing community
   b. employers of gerontological nurses
   c. the gerontological nurse
   d. society

9. Holistic nursing care is concerned with:
   a. the client's physical, mental, social, and spiritual health
   b. the promotion of alternative medical practices
   c. the use of noninvasive rather than technological interventions
   d. modalities to extend life

10. State five slang terms or phrases that are used by the general public to describe older adults.

    Examples: old goat, old crank, old geezer, dirty old man, pops, Grandma Moses, gramps, old hag

CHAPTER 2

Facts About the Aging Population

Chapter 2 surveys a variety of data regarding the older population in an effort to separate myths from realities and to enable the gerontological nurse to establish a foundation for practice based on fact. Tables are plentiful to provide statistical evidence for the generalizations made.

The growth of the older population is presented, with emphasis on an increased life expectancy resulting in more people not only surviving to old age but also spending more time in their senior years than did previous generations. The trend toward a growth in the "old-old" population is discussed. Differences in life expectancy between the sexes and races are shown.

The financial profile of the elderly is reviewed. The point is made that although the percentage of elderly living below the poverty level has steadily decreased, there are disparities between men and women and between the black and white populations.

The increasing educational achievement of the older population is shown with attention to the fact that the trend is toward future senior citizens being better educated than seniors of previous generations.

A discussion of the incidence and prevalence of health problems acquaints the student with the realities of illness in the elderly, emphasizing the major problem of chronic illnesses for this population. Causes of death are listed with attention to heart disease, cancer, and stroke as being the major killers of this group. Related to this is a description of the elderly's use of resources. A brief introduction to the fiscal impact of service utilization by the elderly is offered to stimulate the student to consider broader issues that affect gerontological practice. The challenge is offered to gerontological nurses to demonstrate leadership in ensuring that fiscal constraints do not jeopardize the quality of services for the elderly.

■ Significant Displays, Tables, and Figures

People 65 Years of Age and Older Living Alone (Table 2-6)
Years of School Completed by Age (Table 2-7)
Rates of Acute Illness in Adults by Age (Table 2-8)
Rates of Chronic Illness in Adults by Age (Table 2-9)
Leading Causes of Death for Persons 65 Years of Age and Older (Table 2-10)
Average Length of Hospital Stay (Table 2-11)
Health Insurance Coverage for Persons Age 65 Years and Over (Table 2-12)

STUDENT OBJECTIVES

After reading this chapter, the student should be able to:

1. Describe characteristics of today's elderly population in regard to:

life expectancy	education
gender, race differences	acute and chronic illness
marital status	causes of death
living arrangements	health insurance coverage

2. Discuss projected changes in future generations of elders.

■ Classroom Teaching-Learning Strategies

1. Discuss the fairness and inequity of use by the elderly of a disproportionate amount of government funds for social and health care needs.

2. Discuss factors that contribute to differences in life expectancy, income, and living arrangements between older men and women and between older whites and blacks.

3. Ask the students to discuss changes they can predict in future generations of elders based on statistical trends and the service needs that may be different as a result of changes.

■ Guidelines for Evaluating Critical Thinking Exercises

1.
   - greater numbers of "old-old"; need for nursing services for persons with disease, disability, and dependency
   - large portion of population over age 65, aging of baby boomers; increased need for gerontological nursing services, services will need to be modified to accomodate baby boomers
   - more informed consumers who will want active role in health care
   - growing number of minorities; nursing must be sensitive to cultural diversity in care

2.
- women outlive men and often suffer reduction in income when spouse dies
- women likely to live alone and not have spouse available for caregiving

3. Older black Americans have a lower life expectancy than white Americans and tend to have poorer health and lower economic status.

■ Test Questions

1. The longest life expectancy in the United States is enjoyed by:
   a. white males
   b. black males
   c. white females
   d. black females

2. A true statement regarding poverty in late life is that:
   a. the number of elderly living in poverty has steadily decreased
   b. older men are more likely to be poor than are older women
   c. in late life, poverty rates between white and black groups are similar
   d. more elderly live in poverty now than ever before in history

3. The leading cause of death in the over-65 population is:
   a. cancer
   b. cerebrovascular accident
   c. Alzheimer's disease
   d. heart disease

4. In projecting population trends you could accurately state that:
   a. more people will be spending greater numbers of years in old age
   b. people will be enjoying a longer life span than did previous generations
   c. life expectancies between the sexes and between the races will be similar
   d. the elderly will constitute a smaller percentage of the total population

5. What percentage of the total population do the elderly constitute?
   a. less than 5%
   b. more than 12%
   c. 20%
   d. nearly 50%

6. True or false: As compared with past generations, more people are achieving age 65 today, but they are not living significantly longer after they do.

   a. true

   b. false

7. The most typical living arrangement for an older man would be to live:

   a. alone

   b. in an institution

   c. with a spouse

   d. with a child

8. In comparing acute and chronic illnesses in late life, an accurate statement would be that:

   a. chronic diseases increase and acute illnesses decrease with age

   b. chronic diseases decrease and acute illnesses increase with age

   c. both acute and chronic conditions increase with age

   d. the rate of acute and chronic conditions remains consistent throughout life

9. Most hospital care for persons over age 65 years is paid by:

   a. private insurances

   b. Medicaid

   c. Medicare

   d. self-pay

10. The percentage of the older population institutionalized at any given time is less than:

   a. 5%

   b. 10%

   c. 25%

   d. 50%

CHAPTER 3

Theories of Aging

This chapter begins with a reflection of the interest through the ages in the mystery of aging and brings the student to the present day. Whereas past interest was motivated in discovering immortality, today's interest in understanding the aging process is fueled by a desire to find ways to keep people healthy and active for more years. Students are cautioned that aging theories offer varying degrees of universality, validity, and reliability and that the exact cause of aging remains a mystery.

Major biological theories of aging are presented that attempt to explain the physiological changes experienced through the years. The role of genetic factors in aging is seen in several theories: that people are born with a genetic program that dictates life expectancy, that aging results from self-perpetuating genetic mutations, that aging occurs because of the body's failure to produce a growth substance required for cell growth and reproduction. The cross-link theory proposes that cellular division is threatened as a result of the accumulation of cross-linking agents on the DNA strand. Free radicals are hypothesized to cause physical decline of the body by replacing healthy molecules with faulty ones that create genetic disorder. The accumulation of the "age-pigment" lipofuscin is believed to have a role in the aging process similar to that of free radicals.

Autoimmune reactions as a factor in aging have attracted interest due to the reduction in immunologic function that is seen with age; autoimmune reactions may be associated with the body misidentifying aged cells as foreign agents and attacking them, or misinterpreting normal body constituents due to a breakdown of the immunochemical memory system. The effects of normal wear and tear and stress on the body are viewed as having some influence on causing the body to function less efficiently with age. Although no conclusive evidence exists to link pathogens with age-related declines, longer life expectancies have been realized since disease-causing organisms have been controlled; therefore, disease processes are viewed to have a role in aging. Neuroendocrines and neurochemicals are mentioned due to increased theorization of the relationship of the endocrine gland to the aging process. The premature aging of skin exposed to ultraviolet light and laboratory research with animals have led to the theory that radiation may induce cellular changes that promote aging. Excesses and deficiencies of nutrients have long been and continue to be considered to have a major impact on the aging process. Last, but not least, environmental factors that are known health threats are also believed to influence aging. Students are challenged to consider how information about elements known to affect the aging process can be incorporated into health practices to promote a positive aging experience.

Several psychological theories of aging attempt to explore mental processes, behaviors, and feelings of aging people and to offer insights into mechanisms people use to meet the challenges faced with advancing years. The disengagement theory, although no longer popular or valid, is discussed to acquaint students with the premise of the theory and to demonstrate problems with research of the past; this theory suggests that aging individuals and society withdraw from each other for mutual benefit. The activity theory shifted thinking to the opposite extreme in proposing that older adults should stay in the mainstream of society and be held to the same expectations and norms as middle-aged persons. Although meritorious in some respects, the activity theory proved to lack universality in that the pattern was not appropriate for all individuals. A reasonable compromise was found in the continuity or developmental theory, which stated that personality and basic patterns of behavior are consistent through the lifespan. This theory recognized the complexities of aging in allowing many individual patterns among older adults. Erik Erikson, Robert Peck, Robert Butler, and Myrna Lewis are among the theorists who have described the developmental tasks that must be mastered for healthy psychological aging.

Students are challenged to consider the interrelatedness and interdependence of biological, psychological, and social processes of aging and to be open-minded in their selection of theories to guide their practice.

■ Significant Displays, Tables, and Figures

Erikson's Developmental Tasks (Table 3-1)
Assisting Individuals in Meeting the Psychosocial Challenges of Aging (Display 3-1)
Factors Contributing to a Long and Healthy Life (Display 3-2)

STUDENT OBJECTIVES

After reading this chapter, the student should be able to:

1. Discuss the change in focus regarding learning about factors that influence aging.

2. List the major biological theories of aging.

3. Describe the major psychological theories of aging.

4. Identify factors that promote a healthy aging process.

■ Classroom Teaching-Learning Activities

1. Ask the students to survey current popular literature regarding the themes of healthy aging, staying young, and longevity and to discuss theories that are suggested in them.

2. Discuss health practices that promote healthy aging based on factors considered in the theories of aging.

3. Review nursing actions for helping older adults meet psychological challenges (see Display 3-1).

■ Guidelines for Evaluating Critical Thinking Exercises

1.
- cancer
- autoimmune disorders
- infections

2.
- reduce water and air pollution
- control overcrowded living conditions
- encourage parks and other "green areas"

3.
- sites for housing and health care facility construction
- intergenerational programs in schools, churches, clubs
- public areas that are user-friendly for persons with disabilities

4.
- compile a scrapbook
- guide through an oral history (life review)
- encourage sharing of past events that were meaningful
- recognize past accomplishments
- offer meaningful activities

■ Test Questions

1. The continuity theory states that:
   a. older adults need to be continuously involved with other age groups
   b. the elderly should continue a middle-aged lifestyle
   c. **psychological patterns are consistent through the life span**
   d. life's challenges must be faced and overcome at all ages

2. Lipofuscin influences aging by:

   a. interfering with the diffusion and transport of essential molecules in the cells

   b. causing an accumulation of fatty acids that block vessels and ultimately destroy cells

   c. damaging DNA due to their highly reactive nature

   d. impairing normal immune functions

3. The compression of mortality refers to:

   a. achieving immortality

   b. hastening death

   c. finding everlasting youth

   d. postponing the onset of disease

4. Changes in collagen that reduce tissue elasticity are hypothesized to be related to:

   a. cross-linking

   b. free radicals

   c. lipofuscin

   d. genetic factors

5. Peck's description of body transcendence versus body preoccupation refers to:

   a. achieving satisfaction through the reflection of the past rather than being preoccupied with the limited amount of years remaining

   b. finding psychological pleasures rather than becoming focused on health problems or age-related limitations

   c. developing satisfactions from one's identity as a person rather than through the work role

   d. preparing for death by going into altered states of consciousness as a coping mechanism for physical impairments

6. Free radicals are:

   a. damaging to proteins, enzymes, and DNA

   b. molecules that injure collagen

   c. antibodies that influence autoimmune reactions

   d. fat-protein byproducts of metabolism

7. True or false: One autoimmune theory of aging hypothesizes that the body begins to perceive aging cells as foreign to the body and forms antibodies to destroy them.

   a. true

   b. false

8. An older client asks about the role of nutrition and aging and for your recommendations. Your best advice would be to suggest that she:

   a. take a daily anti-oxidant supplement

   b. eliminate meat from her diet

   c. take vitamin E and bee pollen supplements

   d. eat a well-balanced diet

9. All of the following are valid criticisms of the disengagement theory except:

   a. it allows for unique responses to aging

   b. the population studied to develop the theory was not a representative sample

   c. many older adults do not wish to withdraw from society

   d. society can be deprived of the contributions of older persons

10. Describe at least three actions to assist older adults in meeting developmental tasks of aging.

    Reminiscence, oral histories, compiling scrapbooks/photo albums

CHAPTER 4

Cultural Diversity

Chapter 4 presents some of the unique health attitudes and practices among major ethnic groups in the United States to assist the student in gaining a sensitivity toward nursing people of diverse cultural backgrounds.

The chapter begins with a general discussion of immigration, emphasizing that values and customs are deeply ingrained and have not been erased upon entry into a new country. Although general characteristics are reviewed, the student is advised to avoid stereotyping groups.

Black Americans are composed primarily of persons of African descent, although persons immigrating from Haiti, Tahiti, and Jamaica also are included. Vast differences can exist among black persons from various countries, as well as among black Americans from different regions of this country. Life expectancy is lower among blacks as compared with whites, although survival of the two populations balances after the seventh decade of life (cross-over phenomenon). The health status of black Americans is poorer than that of their white cohorts. Some of the clinical differences in the presentation of symptoms are reviewed.

Native Americans are discussed. This group consists of 493 tribes that can represent an estimated 250 different Native American languages. Health status is related to good and evil forces or rewards and punishment of behaviors. Harmony with nature is important, and nontraditional health practices are common. Special rituals may be used during sickness and death. Elders are respected.

Although not an ethnic group per se, Jewish Americans are included in the chapter because of their unique identity and beliefs. Strong family bonds and positive feelings toward the elderly are common among Jews. Religious traditions that affect health practices and service delivery (e.g., kosher diet, restrictions practiced by Orthodox Jews) are presented.

More than 10 million Asian Americans reside in the United States and are a growing minority of elders. Chinese Americans and their high regard of the aged are discussed. There is a discussion of some of the basics of traditional Chinese medicine, such as the balance of yin and yang, herbs, acupuncture, and acupressure. Like the Chinese, Japanese Americans share a respect for their elders and utilize many traditional practices that may be considered nonconventional in this country. Fillipinos, Koreans, Vietnamese, and Cambodians are other Asian groups included in this discussion.

Spaniards, Mexicans, Cubans, and Puerto Ricans are among the groups considered Hispanic. To many members of this group, English is a second language. Prayer and the use of traditional practitioners for the management of health problems are common. The elderly are held in high esteem.

The chapter ends with a discussion of the implications of cultural diversity for nursing practice. Suggestions for eliciting life stories are included with emphasis that this is a powerful tool to learn about cultural influences. The student is urged to respect, learn about, and incorporate unique characteristics and practices of diverse cultures into nursing care activities.

■ Significant Displays, Tables, and Figures

Chinese Medicine (Display 4-1)
Eliciting Life Stories (Display 4-2)

■ Student Objectives

After reading this chapter, the student should be able to:

1. Describe the unique views of health and attitudes toward the aged of these major groups:
Black Americans
Native Americans
Jewish Americans
Asian Americans
Hispanic Americans

2. Identify ways in which nursing care may need to be modified to accommodate persons of diverse ethnic backgrounds.

■ Classroom Teaching-Learning Activities

1. Ask the students to interview their own families for insights into their immigration experience, cultural practices, and attitudes toward the aged, and to discuss their findings.

2. Discuss problems that may be encountered in nursing practice as a result of cultural differences and strategies that can be used to prevent and correct them.

3. Ask the students to locate churches and ethnic-related organizations in the community that could be helpful to the health care team in service delivery to persons with specific ethnic backgrounds.

■ Guidelines for Evaluating Critical Thinking Exercises

1.
   - Black Americans: strong family ties, history of prejudicial treatment, poor health status
   - Native Americans: traditional healing measures may be used, may be distrustful of U.S. health care system
   - Jewish Americans: Sabbath and holidays, kosher dietary practices
   - Asian Americans: may use traditional Chinese medicine, view health as balance of yin/yang
   - Hispanic Americans: strong family ties, may not be fluent in English, prayer and family caregiving popular

2.
   - native healing practices may need to be sustituted for conventional medical treatments
   - ethnic foods need to be considered in planning special diets
   - interpreters may be needed
   - care may need to be withheld during Sabbath/holidays
   - special efforts may be needed to learn about unique cultural background and practices

■ Test Questions

1. Which is a valid statement about black elders in America?

   a. **They have a lower rate of institutionalization compared with white elders.**

   b. Their life expectancy is now similar to the white population.

   c. Societal prejudices have resulted in weak family bonds.

   d. They depend on government agencies rather than family for assistance.

2. Which of the following would be unnecessary in offering a kosher diet to an Orthodox Jew?

   a. not serving meat and milk products at the same meal

   b. not serving meat and milk products from the same dishes

   c. **prohibiting women from pouring milk in men's glasses**

   d. eliminating shellfish from all meals

3. The energy forces of yin and yang are associated with:
    a. medicine men's healing rituals
    b. traditional Chinese medicine
    c. trances induced by Sobadoras
    d. Issei healing practices

4. The cross-over phenomenon refers to:
    a. the shedding of traditional ethnic beliefs
    b. assimilation of practices of the new country
    c. the rapid decline in health status that occurs when one replaces traditional ethnic practices with the conventional ones of the new country
    d. the similarity in life expectancy that occurs between white and black elders after they reach their seventh decade

5. In predicting the cultural profile of future populations of elders, it would be accurate to say:
    a. greater diversity will be apparent
    b. there will be little difference among various groups
    c. few individuals will speak a language other than English
    d. full assimilation will be completed

6. A valid statement about Native Americans is that they:
    a. can belong to one of 12 recognized tribes
    b. look to health care professionals to make health-related decisions for them
    c. may use spiritual rituals, medicine men, and herbal remedies
    d. are characterized by a large percentage of older adult members

7. True or false: Black elderly have a higher rate of institutionalization than white elderly.
    a. true
    b. false

8. *Issei* is the term to describe:
    a. Hispanic midwives and healers
    b. Chinese physicians
    c. one who has left the Native American way of life
    d. first-generation Japanese Americans

9. A Jewish client asks you to avoid making a home visit during his Sabbath. To honor this request you would not schedule your visits:

   a. from sundown Friday to sundown Saturday

   b. from sundown Friday to sunrise Sunday

   c. all day Sunday

   d. during the day on Friday

10. A nurse friend tells you that the long-term care facility in which she works celebrates St. Patrick's Day, Black History Month, Hanukkah, and other holidays of ethnic groups represented by the resident population. You understand that this practice is:

    a. advantageous to the residents

    b. in violation of federal law

    c. offensive to the residents

    d. demoralizing to the residents

CHAPTER 5

Life Transitions

Chapter 5 explores the many losses and changes faced by aging individuals and nursing's role in helping clients cope with these challenges.

Family changes are reviewed with special emphasis on the changes in the parental role. Pros and cons of having children become independent adults are discussed. The normal pattern for the elderly to be involved and have regular contact with their children is described.

The concept of ageism is discussed. Common misperceptions are listed to prepare the student to react to some of the real prejudice that may be confronted. Erikson's developmental stages (introduced in Chapter 4) are reinforced with a discussion of factors that contribute to integrity versus despair in the last stage of the life cycle.

The grandparenting role is reviewed, highlighting the new challenges to today's grandparents that have resulted from changes in family structures and activities. Issues discussed include the impact of working mothers of minor children, homosexual parents, step-families, new profiles of grandparents, and children being raised by grandparents.

The common experience in late life of widowhood is described along with its many ramifications. Suggestions are offered as to ways in which the nurse can assist widowed persons in adjusting to this new role.

The major adjustment of retirement is discussed. Emphasis is made as to the difficulty in becoming a retiree in a society in which the work ethic and occupational identity are so important. Atchley's classic phases of retirement are outlined, and nursing interventions for each phase are offered.

Although a later chapter is devoted to death and dying, the issue of death is presented in terms of the acute awareness of mortality felt in late life. The role of the gerontological nurse in assisting elders in life review and leaving legacies to the young is suggested.

The impact of physical aging on psychosocial well-being is discussed. Related nursing interventions are provided, such as providing education, promoting optimal function, and offering assistance as needed.

Economic realities are described. The problems arising from limited income in late life are reviewed. The student is challenged to be aware of the impact of economic welfare on health status and to advocate for adequate income for this group.

The increasing difficulty of remaining socially involved as one ages is discussed. Resources that can aid older adults are described. The differences between being alone and being lonely are reviewed.

■ Significant Displays, Tables, and Figures

Nursing Diagnosis Highlight: Altered Role Performance
Retirement Budget (Table 5-1)

■ Student Objectives

After reading this chapter, the student should be able to:

1. Discuss changes that occur in aging families.

2. List challenges faced by widows.

3. Outline the phases of retirement.

4. Discuss the impact of age-related changes on roles.

5. Describe changes in one's social world with aging.

6. List nursing measures to assist individuals in adjusting to the changes and losses of aging.

■ Classroom Teaching-Learning Activities

1. Guide the students in developing a plan for teaching adults between the ages of 20 and 40 years activities in which they should engage to optimize their physical, emotional, and socioeconomic well-being in old age.

2. Discuss the impact on physical health of the multiple losses for which the elderly are at risk.

3. Ask the students to survey popular literature, movies, and television shows for the way in which older adults are portrayed and discuss their findings.

4. Ask the students to identify resources to assist elderly individuals with social and financial needs.

■ Guidelines for Evaluating Critical Thinking Exercises

1. Advantages today's 30-year-old woman may have over her grandmother's generation:
   • more independent; may be better prepared to cope with realities
   • improved financial status due to likelihood of work history
   • improved health status due to increased preventive health care

Disadvantages today's 30-year-old may have compared with her grand-mother's generation:

- may be subjected to stress-related illnesses due to highly stressful lifestyle
- higher divorce rates may cause her to age without a spouse
- may face longer period of parent care

2.

- people are introduced and described in social circles by occupation
- stereotypes are attached to certain work roles

3.

- assist in outlining projected budget
- counsel about health risks and how to minimize them
- provide information on housing options, insurance
- stimulate discussion of developing interests separate from work role

4. Solitude:

- is chosen
- is satisfying and not distressful

Social isolation

- is not desired
- creates stress, depression, anxiety, or other negative reaction

5. Students could review popular television programs, movies, and advertisements for examples.

6.

- promote optimum health status through health education, screening programs, counseling
- introduce topics that should be considered in pre-retirement planning
- encourage the development of interests outside work role
- offer or arrange pre-retirement educational programs
- conduct discussion groups
- refer to community resources

▪ Test Questions

1. The reality about extended families is that they:

   a. were more prevalent in the past

   b. were more myth than fact

   c. are more prevalent today than ever

   d. presented more problems than assistance to family members

2. Eighty-year-old Mrs. Brown is widowed and laments about "losing additional friends all the time." She sighs and questions whether her life had meaning. The nurse's best response is to:

   a. ignore the comment

   b. suggest Mrs. Brown develop new interests

   c. ask Mrs. Brown to describe her past experiences

   d. refer Mrs. Brown for counseling

3. During which phase of retirement does preparation to leave one's job and fantasizing about retirement occur?

   a. reorientation

   b. honeymoon

   c. disenchantment

   d. near

4. Which is a true statement regarding retirement income?

   a. Social Security is the primary means of income for most elderly.

   b. Most retirees have some type of private pension income.

   c. In retirement, the elderly earn at least 75% of what they earned while employed.

   d. A majority of the elderly have no pension and live in poverty.

5. Which is the strongest asset older widows have?

   a. marketable skills

   b. competitive education

   c. other widows

   d. financial independence

6. Reminiscence can:

   a. promote depression by contrasting past to current status

   b. limit the ability of the older adult to enjoy the present

   c. allow the older adult to ignore harsh realities of the present

   d. help the older adult find satisfaction through the life history

7. According to Erikson, satisfaction with one's life history can result in:
   a. integrity
   b. industry
   c. trust
   d. autonomy

8. List three strategies nurses can use to improve role performance of older adults.

9. True or false: Reminiscence is a phenomenon unique to Western society.
   a. true
   b. false

10. Discuss the therapeutic value of solitude.

CHAPTER 6

Common Aging Changes

Chapter 6 surveys the impact of aging on physical and mental health in an effort to equip the student with facts to understand common aging changes. It begins with general changes to the body, such as the reduction in functional cells, intracellular fluid, and subcutaneous fat. The visible outcomes of these general changes are noted in a bonier appearance to the body, baggy eyelids, loss of height, and reduction in body temperature.

The chapter moves on to consider each body system separately, starting with the cardiovascular system. In the absence of pathology, heart size does not change. Valves do become thick and rigid, vessels lose some of their elasticity, and cardiac output is reduced. The longer-lasting tachycardia following added stress on the heart and higher normal blood pressures are discussed for the student's appreciation of differences to consider in assessing vital signs.

The various structural changes to the lungs and chest that affect respiratory activity are reviewed. The lungs expand and expel air less efficiently; residual volume is increased, vital capacity and maximum breathing capacity are reduced, basilar inflation is insufficient, and accumulated or foreign matter in the lung is more difficult to expel. The student is cautioned about the profound effects of immobility on older lungs and the high risk for infections.

The description of changes to the gastrointestinal system begins with emphasis that tooth loss is not a normal outcome of aging; factors contributing to the poor dental status of many elderly are offered. Changes throughout the system are discussed, including reductions in taste sensations, the volume of saliva produced, salivary ptyalin, gastric acids, esophageal motility, gastric emptying time, liver size, and absorption of specific nutrients.

Urinary tract changes that result in urinary frequency, less effective concentration of urine, altered tubular reabsorption of glucose, and stress incontinence are presented. Reproductive system changes are described with mention of the fact that these changes do not equate with a loss of sexual function.

A review of the musculoskeletal system's changes is provided. Muscle mass, strength, and movements are decreased, tendons shrink and harden, reflexes are less acute, and bones become more brittle. The high risk for fractures in the elderly is noted.

Changes to the brain are described, highlighting that these structural changes do not appear to affect thinking and behavior. The changes in the sleep–wake cycle are mentioned, in that stages III and IV of sleep become less prominent.

The inefficiency of each of the five senses is discussed, and the impact of specific changes on sensory function is outlined.

The variety of changes to the endocrine system are reviewed, including the lower basal metabolic rate that results from decreased thyroid gland activity. Changes in hormonal secretion that are mentioned include reductions in thyroid-stimulating hormone, thyroxine, adrenocorticotropic hormone, glucocorticoids, 17-ketosteroids, progesterone, estrogen, testosterone, and luteinizing hormone. Factors contributing to higher blood glucose levels are discussed.

The depressed immune response in late life is described with the review of changes to the immune system with age. Implications for immunization and recognition of inflammatory response are considered.

Differences in thermoregulation are highlighted, including lower mean body temperature, reduced ability to respond to cold temperatures, and different responses to heat.

Integumentary system changes are discussed with mention that diet, health, activity, exposure, and hereditary factors influence the status of the skin in late life. In addition to skin changes, other changes to this system are noted, including thinning and graying of the hair, hardening and slower growth of fingernails, and reduction in perspiration.

The presentation of psychological changes is launched with the interrelatedness of physical, psychological, and social factors. The consistency of the personality over the life span in emphasized. Slower retrieval of memory not regularly used, a decline in fluid intelligence, and a decrease in vigilance performance are changes noted.

Table 6-1 outlines major age-related changes and nursing actions to consider for each and provides a quick summary of changes discussed throughout the chapter. Practical tips for enhancing memory and learning in elders are presented in Tables 6-1 and 6-2.

■ Significant Displays, Tables, and Figures

STUDENT OBJECTIVES

After reading this chapter, the student should be able to:

1. List common age-related changes to the:
   cardiovascular system
   respiratory system
   gastrointestinal system
   genitourinary system
   musculoskeletal system
   nervous system
   sensory organs
   endocrine system
   immune system

2. Describe psychological changes experienced with age.

3. Discuss risks and nursing considerations associated with age-related changes.

■ Classroom Teaching-Learning Activities

1. Ask the students to identify individuals in each of the age ranges of 20–30, 30–40, 40–50, 50–60, 60–70, 70–80, and 80+ and to describe age-related characteristics of each.

2. Discuss factors that can positively and negatively affect the aging process.

3. Outline content for a health education program for senior citizens that reviews normal aging.

4. Discuss risks to health and safety that are increased as a result of age-related changes.

■ Guidelines for Evaluating Critical Thinking Exercises

1. Signs related to normal aging: adding salt to food to compensate for reduced taste sensations; difficulty hearing due to presbycusis (although it is useful to emphasize that this does not occur in nonindustrialized societies)

   Signs attributed to pathology: weight loss, shortness of breath, urinary symptoms, reduced mobility, personality changes, COPD, varicosities, hemorrhoids

Factors that contributed to his health conditions

- occupation: truck driving (urinary symptoms, varicosities)
- smoking

Risks and nursing measures to minimize them

- pneumonia, lung cancer: counsel in smoking cessation, teach deep-breathing exercises
- malnutrition: obtain medical treatment for acute conditions, refer for nutrition counseling
- peripheral vascular disease: encourage ambulation and exercises to lower extremities
- skin breakdown: encourage mobility and frequent position changes, counsel in reduction of sodium intake
- social isolation: obtain audiometric evaluation, encourage socialization, refer to senior citizen centers

2. Discussion of age-related changes students note in themselves and their parents.

3.

- engage in regular exercise
- remain physically and mentally active
- don't smoke or abuse drugs and alcohol
- follow good nutritional practices
- drink at least 1200 mL of water daily
- obtain regular preventive health checkups
- get symptoms/changes evaluated promptly
- avoid exposure to pollutants
- control stress

■ Test Questions

1. Cardiovascular changes are most frequently noted:
   a. as a result of interruptions to sleep
   b. in the early morning when activity is initiated
   c. during periods of extended inactivity or immobility
   d. when added demands are placed on the heart

2. One of the reasons aspiration in the elderly is a significant risk is because:

    a. their gag reflex is absent

    b. esophageal emptying is delayed

    c. gastric motility and emptying time are increased

    d. the esophagus becomes constricted

3. Changes in the genitourinary system include all of the following except:

    a. loss of sexual function

    b. reduced concentration of urine

    c. urinary frequency

    d. urinary retention

4. Which is a valid statement regarding learning in late life?

    a. After a longer early phase the older adult is able to keep pace with younger individuals.

    b. Older people show no difference in the performance of perceptual motor tasks as compared with younger persons.

    c. There is a tendency for the elderly to analyze data rather than rely on simple association.

    d. With age there is improvement in the performance of perceptual motor tasks.

5. Which of the following signs would you consider an abnormality in an older adult?

    a. urinary frequency

    b. decreased tendon jerks

    c. yellowing of the lens

    d. tooth loss

6. True or false: Total body fat as a proportion of the body's total composition decreases with age.

    a. true

    b. false

7. The aging respiratory system is characterized by:

    a. ineffective inhalation

    b. reduced residual volume

    c. insufficient basilar inflation

    d. increased maximum breathing capacity

8. The most profoundly reduced taste sensation with age is for which type of flavor?

   a. sweet

   b. salt

   c. bitter

   d. sour

9. True or false: There is a reduction in height with age due to a shrinkage of the long bones of the body.

   a. true

   b. false

10. Which of the following visual findings is not associated with normal aging?

    a. night blindness

    b. yellowing of lens

    c. presbyopia

    d. arcus senilis

UNIT II

Health and Wellness

After reviewing general facts about the aging population, the aging experience, and principles of nursing the aged, *Gerontological Nursing* begins examining specific nursing interventions that can be used to promote health and wellness in older adults. Orem's Self-Care Model provides the theoretical framework for the discussion. Chapters reviewing each of the universal life demands examine the manner in which aging affects the satisfaction of the demand and present interventions that nurses can use to promote and maintain self-care capacity or to assist clients when self-care limitations exist. Due to the high prevalence of medication use among the older population and the self-care responsibilities faced by older adults in administering and monitoring drugs, the chapter on Safe Medication Use is included in this section.

Chapter 7, Facilitating Health, Wellness, and Self-Care, sets the tone for Unit II. A basic introduction to Orem's Self-Care Theory is offered with modifications by the author. The premise is that all human beings face basic needs, or universal life demands, that must be satisfied to be healthy and well. The student is guided to consider the satisfaction of these needs as a primary level of assessment. When a deficit in satisfying a need exists, a second level of assessment is necessary, namely, the determination of which requisite for meeting the demand is at the root of the problem. The student is assisted in viewing the way in which this self-care model is applicable to nursing the well and the ill aged.

The examination of nursing interventions to help older adults meet self-care needs begins in Chapter 8, Ventilation and Circulation. Factors that alter tissue perfusion are discussed with specific nursing measures to improve circulation. Methods to improve breathing effectiveness and prevent respiratory complications are included.

An overview of the manner in which aging affects nutritional status is offered in Chapter 9, Nutrition. Included are the components of a comprehensive nutritional examination and signs of common nutritional problems, such as dehydration and oral health problems. The special nutritional needs of aging women are discussed as a new feature to this edition. Suggestions are offered for minimizing threats to good nutrition in late life.

Elimination of wastes through the bladder, bowel, and skin is reviewed in Chapter 10, Excretion. Specific problems of the elderly in relation to elimination, such as chronic laxative use and fecal impaction, are described. The unique bathing needs of the elderly to accommodate age-related skin changes are discussed.

Chapter 11, Activity and Exercise, considers the difficulty older adults can face in being active and exercises that the elderly can incorporate into their daily lives to promote activity, along with adjustments and precautions. The benefits of mental activity also are discussed. The hazards of inactivity are presented to sensitize the student to the importance of promoting an active state. The presentation of age-related differences in sleep highlights special challenges to the aged in achieving adequate rest; alternatives to sedatives are discussed. The effects of health on physical and mental health and measures to manage stress are included in this chapter.

Chapter 12, Sleep and Rest, reviews age-related differences in sleep stages and natural means to induce sleep. Health conditions associated with altered sleep patters, such as sleep apnea, are described. A discussion of pain control is offered that includes nonpharmacologic approaches to pain management. The issue of stress management is considered.

The importance of achieving a balance of solitude, in order to retreat, reflect, and refresh, and socialization, in order to be stimulated, experience feelings, and be connected to society, is the focus of Chapter 13, Solitude and Connection. Age-related factors that affect social interaction are described, as are nursing interventions to compensate for these factors. The topic of spirituality is addressed in this chapter, with emphasis on spirituality encompassing more than religion; the therapeutic value of strong spiritual beliefs is reviewed.

The unique risks to health and well-being that advanced age poses are presented in Chapter 14, Safety. Preventive practices to reduce safety risks are described.

The significance of the environment to physical and psychosocial health is described in Chapter 15, Environmental Considerations. The effects of normal aging and disease processes on environmental safety and function are discussed. Factors that make the environment more user-friendly to the elderly are outlined.

Chapter 16, Sexuality and Intimacy, begins by examining stereotypical views on sex and the elderly and ways in which the aged's sexuality is disrespected. Through a discussion of the realities of sexual function in late life and factors that contribute to sexual dysfunction, the student is aided in gaining insight into how sexuality and intimacy can be promoted in the elderly.

Chapter 17, Safe Medication Use, considers the benefits and risks to health and wellness that result from medications. The unique aspects of pharmacokinetics and pharmacodynamics in the aged are discussed. Major drug groups are reviewed in regard to their uses, interactions, precautions, and related nursing considerations. The student is helped to gain insight into measures that can be taken to promote safe drug use.

The final chapter in this unit, Chapter 18, Immunity and Infectious Diseases, examines the major changes in immunologic function that accompany aging and offers suggestions for natural approaches to boosting immunologic health. The unique features of common infections are discussed, as are the risks associated with overuse and misuse of antibiotics.

CHAPTER 7

Facilitating Health, Wellness, and Self-Care

In Chapter 7, a modification of Orem's Self-Care Theory is offered as a framework for gerontological nursing practice. This theory is seen as particularly relevant to gerontological practice because it emphasizes health promotion and independence, suggesting that nursing's role is to assist in maintaining or improving the elder's ability to care for self.

Universal life demands (i.e., basic needs that must be fulfilled to possess health and well-being) are listed; they are:

- ventilation and circulation
- nutrition
- excretion
- activity and exercise
- sleep and rest
- solitude and connection
- safety
- normality

The chapters that follow review these life demands and offer related nursing interventions.

The determination of the degree to which universal life demands are satisfied is the first level of assessment for the nurse. When a deficit in fulfilling a demand exists, the nurse must assess the cause of the deficit so that effective, appropriate nursing actions can be planned. Requisites to meet demands are discussed to give the student insights into the factors that influence demand satisfaction. These requisites are:

- physical, mental, and socioeconomic abilities
- knowledge, experience, and skills
- desire and decision to take action

Self-care capacity is present when life demands are fulfilled; a self-care limitation exists when there is an inability of the individual to independently meet demands. The student is guided to consider that nursing interventions focus on strengthening self-care capacity; nurses only "do for" clients when clients are unable to achieve independence. The intent is that the student will understand that elders shouldn't be robbed of independence for the sake of efficiency or expediency.

Since geriatric nursing involves nursing ill elderly, the application of the self-care model to geriatric nursing practice is described. In addition to consideration of the extent to which universal life demands are met, the nurse also must determine the degree to which illness-imposed demands (e.g., medication administration, special treatments, symptom detection) are satisfied. The requisites for meeting illness-imposed demands are similar to those for meeting life demands. Again, the emphasis is to help the client be independent in meeting needs.

A case example is presented to assist the student in the application of the model. In this case, deficits identified are described as nursing diagnoses. Care plan goals and actions follow. The type of action, consistent with the self-care model terminology, is offered adjacent to the description of the nursing action to reinforce the theory.

▪ Significant Displays, Tables, and Figures

Self-Care Model (Figure 7-1)
Self-Care Model for Geriatric Nursing (Figure 7-2)

STUDENT OBJECTIVES

After reading this chapter, the student should be able to:

1. List universal self-care demands.

2. Discuss requisites for meeting self-care demands.

3. Describe the way in which the self-care model is used in gerontological nursing.

4. List nursing actions that assist older adults in fulfilling universal life demands.

▪ Classroom Teaching-Learning Activities

1. Ask the students to identify an older adult with whom they have had experience and outline the elder's self-care capacities and limitations, using the self-care model format.

2. Describe factors in the community and institutional settings that could threaten the independence of the elderly.

3. Discuss the implications of nurses acting or doing for older adults when these individuals have the capacity for independence.

▪ Guidelines for Evaluating Critical Thinking Exercises

1.
  - relocating from foreign country
  - fighting in world wars
  - surviving the Great Depression

2. The boxed information describing the universal life demands can serve as a guide.

3.
   - gains achieved through depending on others (attention, benefits, qualifications, etc.)
   - fear of harming self

4.
   - promotes independence
   - prevents avoidable decline

5.
   - busy schedules in hospitals or health care facilities that pressure nurses to expedite care by doing for patients rather than allowing time for patient to do for self
   - nurses making caregiving decisions "in best interest of patient"
   - nursing staff fearful of incidents or injury by allowing independence

■ Test Questions

1. Which is not a universal life demand?
   a. ventilation and circulation
   b. normality
   c. safety
   d. medication administration

2. When a deficit in fulfilling a life demand has been identified, the nurse would next:
   a. examine the requisites for meeting the demand
   b. develop goals
   c. act for the client until the client can be independent
   d. implement actions to remove the self-care limitation

3. True or false: Self-care limitations can be eliminated.
   a. true
   b. false

4. True or false: A client can have the physical, mental, and socioeconomic abilities to meet a universal life demand but possess a self-care deficit.

   a. true

   b. false

   For the remaining questions, determine whether the action described is an example of:

   a. acting or doing for

   b. strengthening self-care capacity

   c. minimizing self-care limitation

5. Scheduling care activities to provide rest periods to recover from stress

   a. acting for

6. Rewarding positive behavioral changes

   b. strengthening self-care capacity

7. Facing the hearing-impaired individual and speaking clearly

   c. minimizing self-care limitation

8. Providing medications labels that are in large print and color-coded

   c. minimizing self-care limitation

9. Removing noningestible solutions from the environment of a person with dementia

   a. acting for

10. Instructing the client in deep-breathing exercises

    b. strengthening self-care capacity

CHAPTER 8

Ventilation and Circulation

Chapter 8 reviews factors that affect the good oxygenation of all body cells. Age-related changes and diseases that affect circulation are listed, along with nursing interventions that can promote tissue circulation.

Suggestions to enhance effective breathing are addressed. The prevention of respiratory infection is discussed. Actions that older adults can take to prevent and control infection are included, such as identifying and reporting clinical signs of infection and engaging in breathing exercises.

A review of the nursing diagnosis Ineffective Breathing Pattern is offered.

■ Significant Displays, Tables, and Figures

Deep Breathing Exercises (Figure 8-1)
Aging and Risks to Adequate Ventilation and Circulation (Table 8-1)
Indications of Altered Tissue Perfusion (Display 8-1)

STUDENT OBJECTIVES

After reading this chapter, the student should be able to:

1. List factors that can alter tissue perfusion.

2. Describe nursing measures that could improve circulation.

3. Describe measures to reduce the risk of respiratory infection and other respiratory complications.

■ Classroom Teaching-Learning Activities

1. Discuss measures that could be utilized to promote deep breathing for:
   - bedbound elderly
   - older persons with dementia
   - healthy, community-based elders

2. Develop a patient education program for an older adult who possesses a chronic respiratory disease; implement if possible.

▪ Guidelines for Evaluating Critical Thinking Exercises

1.
- walking and other forms of physical exercise
- yoga, tai chi, and other nontraditional exercises
- avoiding obstructions to circulation (crossing legs, garters) and pressure
- maintaining blood pressure within normal range

2. Allows movement of diagram for maximum area for lung expansion.

3.
- they know their own norm and can detect changes early
- they are empowered to be active participants in care

▪ Test Questions

1. Recommended breathing exercises for the elderly should promote:

   a. inhaling to the count of 1, exhaling to the count of 3

   b. inhaling to the count of 1, exhaling to the count of 1

   c. inhaling to the count of 3, exhaling to the count of 3

   d. inhaling to the count of 3, exhaling to the count of 1

2. An age-related change to the lung that can interfere with adequate ventilation is:

   a. less elastic recoil of lungs during expiration

   b. decreased residual capacity

   c. increased vital capacity

   d. less rigidity of thoracic muscles

3. Altered tissue perfusion can be evidenced by:

   a. warm, flushed skin

   b. loss of hair on extremities

   c. tachycardia

   d. edema

4. All of the following signs can be related to carbon dioxide narcosis except:

   a. profuse perspiration

   b. impaired vision

   c. muscle twitching

   d. elevated blood pressure

5. True or false: Most older adults have some problem with carbon dioxide retention.

   a. true

   b. false

6. True or false: Hypertension is a greater cause of poor circulation than hypotension.

   a. true

   b. false

7. True or false: Fever, chest pain, and cough can appear atypically in older adults and delay the recognition of pneumonia.

   a. true

   b. false

8. True or false: Blood pressures of older adults need to be lower to compensate for poor peripheral circulation.

   a. true

   b. false

9. True or false: Peripheral vessels of older adults have reduced elasticity and resistance.

   a. true

   b. false

10. List at least five causes of altered tissue perfusion.

    cardiovascular disease, diabetes mellitus, cancer, renal failure, blood dyscrasias, medications, edema, immobility, malnutrition

Nutrition

The profound impact of nutrition on health and functional capacity is discussed in Chapter 9. Some of the age-related factors that can affect nutritional status are outlined, including the high prevalence of tooth loss, increased taste threshold, decreased thirst sensations, and decreased colonic peristalsis; potential nursing diagnoses associated with these factors are identified.

The key components of a nutritional assessment are reviewed and include:

- History: general health status, medications, food intake and preferences
- Physical examination: hair, skin, muscle tone and strength, eyes, oral cavity, signs and symptoms
- Biochemical evaluation: blood and urine screening
- Cognition and mood: evaluation, alterations
- Anthropometric measurement: height, weight, triceps skinfold measurement, midarm circumference

Special issues regarding nutritional health in late life are addressed. The significance of adequate hydration and specific challenges of the elderly in achieving a good fluid intake are presented. Oral health, an often overlooked but crucial factor in good nutritional status, is reviewed. The special needs of women are an overdue addition to this text; issues such as the need for older women to reduce fat intake and increase calcium intake are considered. With half of the general public consuming vitamins and other nutritional supplements on a daily basis, the topic of nutritional supplements is included. Risks associated with misuse of vitamin, mineral, and herbal supplements are highlighted.

Specific threats to good nutrition and related nursing interventions are discussed. Topics reviewed include poor appetite, indigestion and food intolerance, constipation, and malnutrition. The student is urged to consider a wide range of services to assist elders in meeting their nutritional needs. The nursing diagnosis Fluid Volume Deficit is featured.

■ Significant Displays, Tables, and Figures

Aging and Risks to Nutritional Status (Table 9-1)
Recommended Daily Allowances for People Over 50 Years of Age (Table 9-2)
Components of the Nutritional Assessment (Display 9-1)

Food Guide Pyramid (Figure 9-1)

Risks Associated with Excess Intake of Selected Vitamins and Minerals (Display 9-2)

Side Effects of Extended or Excessive Use of Selected Herbs (Display 9-3)

Herb–Drug Interactions (Display 9-4)

STUDENT OBJECTIVES

After reading this chapter, the student should be able to:

1. List age-related factors that affect dietary requirements in late life.

2. Describe the components of a comprehensive nutritional assessment.

3. Identify causative factors and signs of dehydration.

4. Describe oral health problems that could influence nutritional status and describe recommended oral hygiene for older adults.

5. List the special nutritional needs of aging women.

6. Outline threats to good nutrition in late life and ways to minimize them.

■ Classroom Teaching-Learning Activities

1. Ask the students to interview several older adults and obtain information about the views the elders hold on good nutritional practices.

2. Ask the students to select an ill, aged individual and review the impact that the person's disease(s) and medication(s) potentially can or actually do have on nutritional status.

3. Discuss the difficulties the following individuals may have in adhering to a good diet. Identify resources and nursing interventions to assist each.

   - a nursing home resident
   - a community-based person living alone

■ Guidelines for Evaluating Critical Thinking Exercises

1.

   - ability to chew, swallow, digest, and metaboize food
   - knowledge of proper diet
   - ability to afford, shop for, and prepare food
   - cognitive ability to recognize need for food, understand healthy diet, seek and consume food
   - appetite, desire to eat

2.
- flossing, tooth brushing, denture care
- importance of regular dental exams
- recognizing signs of oral disease

3.
- Discuss advertisements for dietary supplements, claims made.
- Be familiar with resources that can be used by older consumers; provide education and counseling.

4.
- special diets, restrictions
- symptoms (pain, nausea)
- lack of culturally sensitive diet, favorite foods
- environment (odors, sounds, sights)
- lack of socialization during mealtime

5. Review Display 9-1.

■ Test Questions

1. Which is a valid statement regarding dentures in old age?
   a. Gum changes with age cause tooth loss and the need for dentures in most aging persons.
   b. Dentures will need to be refitted as the individual ages.
   c. Dentures eliminate the need for dentist visits.
   d. There is never a need for dentures.

2. The best locations to assess skin turgor in an older adult are over the:
   a. sternum and forehead
   b. wrists and forearm
   c. eyelids and abdomen
   d. chin and elbow

3. You are told that your older patient has a riboflavin deficiency. Signs that would be consistent with this are:
   a. brownish pigmentation over parts of the body exposed to light
   b. fungus infections of the genitalia and feet
   c. red, scaly areas in the folds around the eyes and between the nose and corner of the mouth
   d. small skin elevations that resemble "goosebumps" over the entire body surface

4. Which is an accurate statement regarding caloric requirements in late life?

   a. Caloric requirements are reduced with age.

   b. Male and female caloric requirements become identical.

   c. Caloric requirements are increased after age 75.

   d. Caloric requirements are unchanged between ages 25 and 75.

5. Which of the following meal plans is the healthiest for an older adult?

   a. skipping breakfast and eating a regular size lunch and dinner

   b. eating the largest meal of the day prior to bedtime

   c. eating three large meals and small supplements in between

   d. eating five small meals throughout the day

6. For the average older adult, what percentage of the total caloric intake should be from dietary fat?

   a. 10

   b. 30

   c. 50

   d. none

7. Of all the following individuals of the same size, who requires the least caloric intake?

   a. 80-year-old woman

   b. 75-year-old man

   c. 45-year-old woman

   d. 65-year-old man

8. List three factors that contribute to the risk of reduced fluid intake in the elderly.

   reduced thirst sensations, physical disabilities that limit ability to obtain and drink fluids, cognitive impairments that reduce ability to recognize need to drink

9. Which of the following practices would you advise an older adult to change?

   a. limiting fried foods

   b. sitting in a high-Fowler's position while eating

   c. lying down and resting immediately following a meal

   d. drinking 1500 mL of fluids daily

10. True or false: A weight loss greater than 5% in a 1-month period of time is significant and warrants evaluation.

    a. true

    b. false

CHAPTER 10

Excretion

The important function of eliminating wastes through the bowel, bladder, and skin is discussed in Chapter 10. The effects of aging on urinary elimination can result in urinary frequency, nocturia, retention, reduced ability to concentrate urine, and alterations in the filtration of substances through the kidneys. Emphasis is given to the fact that incontinence is not a normal outcome of the aging process.

The myth of the need for daily bowel elimination and laxative abuse are discussed. The student is made aware of the risks associated with these issues and of interventions to correct and prevent them. The nursing diagnosis of Constipation is reviewed with care planning goals and actions. Practical hints are offered for the management of flatulence. Signs indicating fecal impaction and related corrective measures are described.

Consumers are increasingly using complementary measures for health promotion, and fasting is one such practice. The benefits, process, and risks associated with fasting are discussed.

Although bathing is viewed as a basic process, there are special concerns in relation to the bathing needs of older adults. Age-related changes reduce bathing needs, and the student is cautioned about the hazardous effects on the skin of excessive bathing. Recommendations for bath water temperature are offered to reduce burn risk.

■ Significant Displays, Tables, and Figures

Aging and Risks to Normal Excretion of Wastes (Table 10-1)
Flatus Bag (Figure 10-1)

STUDENT OBJECTIVES

After reading this chapter, the student should be able to:

1. List age-related changes that affect elimination.

2. Recognize safety risks associated with patterns of urinary elimination in old age.

3. Describe problems associated with chronic laxative use.

4. List measures to facilitate bowel elimination.

5. Identify indications of fecal impaction.

6. Discuss alterations in bathing practices to accommodate age-related skin changes.

7. Discuss the effects of fasting.

■ Classroom Teaching-Learning Activities

1. Discuss measures that could be used to facilitate bowel elimination without the use of laxatives.

2. Ask the students to survey a group of senior citizens to determine the seniors' knowledge base concerning bowel and bladder elimination. Advise the students to provide education as necessary.

■ Guidelines for Evaluating Critical Thinking Exercises

1. Refer to Table 10-1

2. Toileting breaks every 2 hours

3. High-fiber foods, increased fluid intake, regular exercise

4.
- urinary tract infection
- constipation; fecal impaction and hemorrhoids as secondary complications
- falls from stress incontinence

■ Test Questions

1. The most common cause of urinary retention in older men is:
   a. **prostatic hypertrophy**
   b. urinary tract infection
   c. penile strictures
   d. diabetes mellitus

2. Which problem is least likely to be associated with chronic laxative use?
   a. dehydration
   b. depletion of fat-soluble vitamins
   c. electrolyte imbalances
   d. **stress incontinence**

3. Eighty-two-year-old Mrs. Clark presents with abdominal discomfort, a distended abdomen, and diarrhea. You could suspect that her problem most likely is:

   a. colitis

   b. fecal impaction

   c. colon cancer

   d. bowel obstruction

4. Water temperature for bathing older adults should range between:

   a. 80°–85° F

   b. 90°–95° F

   c. 100°–105° F

   d. 120°–125° F

5. An age-related change that affects excretion is:

   a. decreased bladder capacity

   b. increased glomerular filtration rate

   c. decreased nighttime production of urine

   d. increased oil production

6. Which of the following symptoms is least likely to be associated with urinary retention?

   a. urinary frequency

   b. dribbling after voiding

   c. palpable bladder

   d. burning upon urination

7. True or false: Older adults can be hyperglycemic without evidence of glycosuria.

   a. true

   b. false

8. Eighty-two-year-old Mr. Jinks tells you that he "sponges off" each day but only gets into the tub for a complete bath every 4 days. Your best action is to:

   a. do nothing

   b. request someone to bathe him daily

   c. explain to him the importance of daily tub bathing

   d. explore the reasons for his inattention to hygiene

9. True or false: The older adult may require less frequent toileting when in a recumbent position.

   a. true

   b. false

10. If you discovered urinary retention in an older woman, one of the first conditions you would look for is:

    a. prolapsed uterus

    b. fecal impaction

    c. glycosuria

    d. senile vaginitis

CHAPTER 11

Activity and Exercise

This chapter promotes activity as having many physical, psychological, and social benefits and identifies some of the unique problems faced by the elderly as they attempt to be active. Age-related factors that can interfere with activity are listed along with related nursing diagnoses. Special efforts to assist the aged in compensating for these factors are discussed. Guidelines for exercise in late life and associated precautions are presented. The value of incorporating exercise into one's daily routine is promoted. An explanation of t'ai chi and yoga is offered to acquaint the student with the use of unconventional forms of exercise. The nursing diagnosis Impaired Physical Mobility is reviewed, with goals and interventions that nurses can use to assist older persons who possess this problem.

Along with physical activity, the importance of mental stimulation and challenge is discussed. The student is advised to plan mental activity with consideration of the older adult's lifelong interests and patterns.

Hazards of inactivity are described and include changes in physiological function, increased risk of complications, changes in mood and self-concept, increased dependency, and reduced opportunities for socialization.

■ Significant Displays, Tables, and Figures

Aging and Risks to Maintaining an Active State (Table 11-1)
Exercise Program Guidelines for Older Adults (Display 11-1)
Nonconventional Forms of Exercise (Display 11-2)
Deleterious Effects of Inactivity (Display 11-3)
Exercises (Figure 11-3)

STUDENT OBJECTIVES

After reading this chapter, the student should be able to:

1. Discuss factors that interfere with an active state.

2. Describe exercises that would be appropriate for the elderly.

3. Describe sources of mental stimulation for older adults.

4. List adverse effects of inactivity.

■ Classroom Teaching-Learning Activities

1. Discuss age-related changes that affect the ability of the elderly to be active.

2. Show videos demonstrating t'ai chi and yoga exercises. Instruct the students' practice and discuss how these can be used with older adults.

3. Describe activities that can be used to promote mental stimulation in healthy community-based elderly and ill, institutionalized aged.

■ Guidelines for Evaluating Critical Thinking Exercises

1.
   - elders' obstacles to active states: health conditions, limited finances to engage in leisure pursuits, ageism
   - aspects of society that discourage physical activity in elders: fast-paced society, new housing developments often lack walking and public areas for activity, athletic centers can be expensive and prohibitive to elders on fixed incomes, youth-oriented society

2. Students can offer wide variation in discussing this one.

3.
   - mental stimulation for community-based elders: discussion groups, book clubs, classes at local colleges, Internet activities, volunteerism, trips, games, crafts
   - mental stimulation for resident in long-term care facility: discussion groups, speakers, reading, intergenerational activities, games, crafts

4.
   - nurse's expectations can: stimulate activity (self-fulfilling prophecy), demonstrate respect for elder's capabilities, help to identity unique strengths and interests that can be built upon

■ Test Questions

1. True or false: Although it can stimulate circulation, t'ai chi subjects elders to falls.
   a. true
   b. false

2. Which is the best source of physical activity?
   a. exercises that focus on good speed and rhythm
   b. weight lifting at slow speed with high weights
   c. high-level resistance exercises
   d. isometric exercises

3. All of the following can result from inactivity except:
   a. reduced pulse rate
   b. increased blood pressure
   c. increased dependency
   d. demineralization of bones

4. True or false: Elders are at no greater risk of dehydrating during physical exercise than aldults of other ages.
   a. true
   b. false

5. When planning activities for older adults, it is most beneficial to:
   a. provide activities that are new to them
   b. offer equal amounts of individual and group activities
   c. build on past activities and interests
   d. focus on quiet, passive activities

6. Describe three ways in which a chronic disease can affect activity levels.

   Possible answers:
   - inability to move or use body parts
   - cognitive impairments that prohibit ability to follow directions
   - symptoms: pain, fatigue, dizziness, weakness
   - side effects of medications used to treat conditions
   - reduced money to engage in leisure pursuits

7. Which are the best types of exercises for older adults?
   a. resistance exercises
   b. isometric exercises
   c. high-weight, low-repetition exercises
   d. low-weight, high-repetition exercises

8. The nonconventional exercise that combines breathing exercises, meditation, and asanas is:
   a. yoga
   b. t'ai chi
   c. reflexology
   d. imagery

9. List five adverse effects of inactivity.

   Possible answers: muscle atrophy, weakness, joint stiffness, weight gain, postural hypotension, pressure ulcers, constipation, poor digestion, reduced appetite, boredom, depression, social isolation

10. Describe major factors to assess in older adults before initiating an exercise program.

    Refer to Display 11-1.

CHAPTER 12

Sleep and Rest

This chapter provides a listing of factors that interfere with the needs for sleep and rest and suggestions for compensating for them. Safety considerations related to sleep (e.g., side rails, cautious use of sedatives) are described. The student is offered suggestions for measures to promote sleep without the use of sedatives. The nursing diagnosis Sleep Pattern Disturbance is reviewed and provides goals and interventions to assist older adults with this problem.

Stress management is discussed. The student is guided to consider the ill effects of chronic stress. Measures to prevent and control stress are reviewed. In addition to conventional stress management measures, meditation, herbs, guided imagery, and prayer are presented as useful complementary therapies.

■ Significant Displays, Tables, and Figures

Aging and Risks to the Ability to Achieve Rest (Table 12-1)
Stages of Sleep and Late Life Differences (Display 12-1)

STUDENT OBJECTIVES

After reading this chapter, the student should be able to:

1. List differences between younger and older adults in sleep stages.

2. Describe nonpharmacological means to induce sleep.

3. Describe health conditions that could cause altered sleep patterns.

4. Discuss schedules of activity and rest that could benefit elders.

5. List nonpharmacological measures for pain control.

6. List the body's reaction to stress.

7. Describe approaches to reduce stress.

■ Classroom Teaching-Learning Activities

1. Discuss factors in a typical health care facility environment that can interfere with rest and sleep.

2. Demonstrate guided imagery, basic massage techniques, and other measures that can be used by nurses as alternatives to sedatives.

3. Discuss sources of stress in older adults' lives and ways to reduce them.

■ Guidelines for Evaluating Critical Thinking Exercises

1.

- exercise
- guided imagery
- herbal teas, aromatherapy
- warm bath at bedtime
- establishment of regular bedtime

2.

- role changes
- multiple chronic conditions
- ageism
- altered appearance
- reduced income secondary to retirement
- high prevalence of loss/death of peers, widowhood

■ Test Questions

1. The stages of sleep in late life that are less prominent are (more than one answer can be selected):
   a. stage I
   b. stage II
   c. stage III
   d. stage IV

2. Which of the following symptoms is inconsistent with sleep apnea?
   a. snoring
   b. sudden awakening and gasping for breath
   c. one episode of cessation of breathing
   d. daytime fatigue

3. List five reactions to stress.

   Increased mental alertness, cold extremities, conversion of glycogen to glucose, increased heart and respiratory rates, pupil dilation, more acute hearing, increased clotting activity, reduced sexual interest and drive, reduced ability to concentrate, anxiety, fear, increased errors

4. True or false: Administration of a nonnarcotic analgesic with a narcotic could decrease the amount of narcotic that is needed by the older person in pain.

   a. true

   b. false

5. The most deleterious type of stress is:

   a. acute episodic

   b. psychological

   c. physiological

   d. chronic unrelieved

6. Describe nonpharmacological means to promote sleep.

   Possible answers: massage, therapeutic touch, (noncaffeinated) herbal teas, aromatherapy with lavender or valerian, music, some physical activity in early evening, bedtime snack, establishing regular bedtime, limiting caffeine in later part of day

7. True or false: Persons with sleep apnea will be able to breathe most effectively if they sleep in a supine position.

   a. true

   b. false

8. Describe how a stethoscope can be used to facilitate communication with a hearing-impaired person during the night.

   The earpiece can be placed in the person's ear and the caregiver can speak into the diaphragm portion.

9. True or false: Normal aging has less effect on the quantity of sleep than the quality of sleep.

   a. true

   b. false

10. In reference to sleep stages, persons with dementias have:

    a. no stage I and II sleep

    b. heightened REM

    c. no stage IV sleep

    d. all of the above

CHAPTER 13

Solitude and Connection

I n this chapter an effort is made to sensitize the student to the importance of a balance of solitude and social interaction. The benefits of this balance are discussed, as well as age-related factors that threaten it. Communication obstacles that arise from vision and hearing impairments are reviewed. Nursing interventions that facilitate the elderly's ability to socialize are discussed.

A discussion of being alone versus being lonely emphasizes that the elderly's choice to be alone differs from being socially isolated. The nursing diagnosis Social Isolation is highlighted to assist the student in understanding interventions that are beneficial to the socially isolated elder.

A discussion of spirituality is included in this chapter to help the student recognize the importance to older adults of deriving a sense of purpose, hope, and love through this sphere. The difference between religion and spirituality is emphasized. Research supporting the role of faith in health and healing is offered. The student is challenged to guide elders in developing a sense of integrity by balancing the needs of the body, mind, and spirit.

■ Significant Displays, Tables, and Figures

The Role of Faith in Health and Healing (Display 13-1)
Meditation (Display 13-2)
Aging and Risks to Solitude and Social Interaction (Table 13-1)

STUDENT OBJECTIVES

After reading this chapter, the student should be able to:

1. Discuss the importance of a balance of solitude and social interaction in one's life.

2. List communication obstacles resulting from hearing and visual impairments.

3. Describe variables that affect socialization in late life.

4. Differentiate between being alone and loneliness.

5. Discuss the role of spirituality in one's life.

■ Classroom Teaching-Learning Activities

1. Ask the students to interview several older adults and explore the role that religious beliefs/faith has had in their lives.

2. Analyze their community for opportunities for elders to interact with persons of other ages.

3. Discuss ways in which typical health care facilities minimize opportunities for elders to have periods of solitude and suggestions for improving this.

■ Guidelines for Evaluating Critical Thinking Exercises

1.
   - promotes health of elders
   - affords younger generations advantage of elders' experience and wisdom

2.
   - hearing and visual impairments can affect communication
   - physical appearance of advanced age can trigger ageism in interactions
   - fast-paced, youth-oriented society may discourage elders' participation

3. Discuss lack of privacy and tendency of staff to enter patients' rooms whenever they please. Discuss respect for privacy, establishment of "quiet times," use of "Do Not Disturb" signs.

4.
   - What is your source of strength?
   - Do you believe in God or a Higher Power?
   - Would you like to have a visit from clergy?

■ Test Questions

1. You are conducting a group activity with 10 older adults. The best seating arrangement would be to place the chairs:
   a. in two rows of five at perpendicular angles
   b. in two rows of five, classroom style
   c. in a circle
   d. in a straight line

2. Which is an accurate statement regarding periods of solitude for older adults?

   a. **They are therapeutic.**

   b. They imply loneliness.

   c. They are more important than social activity in late life.

   d. They promote depression and other mental health problems.

3. Which of the following is a valid statement regarding religion and spirituality?

   a. Religion and spirituality are one and the same.

   b. **Religion is one aspect of spirituality.**

   c. Religion is a broader concept than spirituality.

   d. Spirituality is a belief system for those who do not have a religious affiliation.

4. Communication with an elder with presbycusis can be enhanced by:

   a. speaking softly and distinctly

   b. facing and shouting slowly

   c. **speaking loudly and clearly**

   d. using sign language

5. The best means to remove cerumen from the ear is by:

   a. **irrigating the ear with gentle pressure**

   b. irrigating the ear with forceful pressure

   c. gently rotating a cotton-tipped applicator in the ear canal

   d. picking the cerumen out with a wire probe

6. True or false: To compensate for poor peripheral vision, the nurse should approach the client from the side rather than the front.

   a. true

   b. **false**

7. True or false: Meditation is an activity that is intended to calm the mind and focus thoughts on the present.

   a. **true**

   b. false

8. True or false: Although most people find them personally beneficial, there is no hard evidence demonstrating that religious practices have any positive effect on health status.

   a. true

   b. **false**

9. Describe three interventions to prevent or reduce social isolation.
   - improvement of health conditions that could impair socialization
   - referral to senior citizen center or activities
   - assistance in obtaining financial assistance, transportation
   - provide "visitor-friendly" environment in health care facilities

10. Describe the impact of self-concept and body image on social interaction.

    Positive self-concept promotes confidence for socialization.

CHAPTER 14

Safety

C hapter 14 begins by reviewing the problem of injuries in the elderly. Although the elderly have an overall lower rate of injury as compared with young adults, older women have a higher rate of injuries than any adult female group; male injury rate declines through the years. Accidents rank as the sixth leading cause of death in the older population.

There is a discussion of age-related factors that can threaten safety, such as sensory alterations, weaker gag reflex, and more fragile skin. The increased prevalence of chronic disease, high volume of medications consumed, and reduced income are among the factors discussed that are more common in late life and increase safety risks.

Preventive practices to reduce safety risks are described and include sufficient fluid intake, vision aids, infection prevention, sensible clothing, wise medication use, environmental safety, crime avoidance, and safe driving. The student is offered suggestions for identifying and correcting problems early, including teaching elders to identify and report changes and abnormalities in their own health status. The nursing diagnosis High Risk for Injury is highlighted.

The special risks associated with physical and mental impairments are discussed. The student is offered specific interventions to protect these individuals.

Falls are a significant concern in gerontological nursing because of their high incidence: approximately 30% of the elderly experience a fall each year. Factors contributing to falls are discussed, as are interventions to prevent and manage falls.

The chapter concludes with a review of measures that can promote safety to compensate for age-related changes and health problems. The student is provided with an environmental checklist that can trigger thinking regarding risk factors in the elder's home.

■ Significant Displays, Tables, and Figures

Incidence of Injuries for Various Age Groups (Table 14-1)
Deaths by Injuries by Gender and Age (Table 14-2)
Aging and Risks to Safety (Table 14-3)
Checklist of Risk Factors for Falls (Display 14-1)
Environmental Checklist (Display 14-2)

STUDENT OBJECTIVES

After reading this chapter, the student should be able to:

1. Describe the effects of aging on safety.

2. List measures to reduce the elderly's risks to safety and well-being.

3. Discuss unique safety risks of individuals with functional impairments.

4. List factors that contribute to falls in the elderly.

5. Describe safety aids that can be of benefit to the elderly.

■ Classroom Teaching-Learning Activities

1. Discuss factors that increase the elderly's risks for injuries.

2. Ask the students to list potential safety hazards to elderly individuals that are present in a public setting, the average home, and a hospital setting.

3. Describe modifications that could be made to the average home to reduce safety hazards for an older individual with a dementia. Ask the students to locate sources for purchasing safety aids that could be used.

■ Guidelines for Evaluating Critical Thinking Exercises

1.

- importance of having health conditions treated and symptoms controlled
- wearing safe clothing and shoes
- home safety pointers
- driving safety pointers

2.

- risks in community: hot water temperature excessively high, poor household maintenance, crime, clutter
- risks in acute hospital: equipment/clutter in pathway, falling out of bed, high activity level 24 hours/day, cold environmental temperatures, solutions left at bedside intended for external use that can be accidentally ingested
- risks in long-term care facility: confused residents, equipment/clutter in pathway, falling out of bed, cold environmental temperatures, solutions left at bedside intended for external use that can be accidentally ingested, lack of timely response to request for assistance

3.

- hypertension: falls
- arthritis: falls, inability to safely operate appliances or close/lock windows and doors
- right-sided weakness: falls, impaired ability to detect items in path, inability to feel pressure/burns/pain
- Alzheimer's disease: drinking noningestible solutions, leaving items on stove unattended, improper use of appliances, falls, scalding in bathtub

4.

- installing lever-shaped door handles and faucet knobs
- controlling hot water temperatures
- replacing fluorescent lighting with several sources of soft lighting
- installing grab bars in bathtub/shower, handrails on stairways
- obtaining emergency call system
- installing tubs and shower stalls with nonslip surfaces
- removing scatter rugs

■ Test Questions

1. Regarding the rate of accidents and injuries in the older population, which is a true statement?
   a. The elderly have the highest death rate from accidents of all age groups.
   b. Older men have a higher rate of injuries than older women.
   c. Accidents rank as the sixth leading cause of death in the elderly.
   d. The elderly have a higher rate of accidents than any age group.

2. True or false: There is no relationship between an older adult's history of falling and current risk of falling.
   a. true
   b. false

3. Which of the following findings in the environment of an older adult could present a safety risk and require correction?
   a. hot water temperature of 105° F
   b. use of contrasting colors from floor surface on stairs
   c. use of a bath stool
   d. electrical outlet 3 feet above bathtub

4. True or false: Older women have a higher rate of injuries than any adult female group.

   a. **true**

   b. false

5. List five age-related factors that increase safety risks for the elderly.

   Decreased peripheral vision, farsightedness, presbycusis, decreased pressure sensations, slower response and reaction time, senile cataracts, higher prevalence of chronic conditions

6. True or false: A fracture may not be apparent immediately after a fall.

   a. **true**

   b. false

For questions 7 to 10, state whether the frequency of vaccination should be:

   a. annually

   b. every 5 years

   c. every 10 years

   d. once in a lifetime

7. Influenza:

   a. **annually**

8. Pneumoccal:

   d. **once in a lifetime**

9. Tetanus:

   c. **every 10 years**

10. Diphtheria:

   c. **every 10 years**

CHAPTER 15

Environmental Considerations

This chapter presents an overview of the purpose of the environment. Maslow's Hierarchy of Needs is used as a framework for demonstrating that the environment meets various levels of needs, from the basic physiological need for shelter through the need for self-actualization.

The impact of age-related changes on environmental health and safety is discussed. Specific effects of sensory changes, common health problems, and drug therapy are listed.

Physical aspects of the environment are reviewed. Examples are offered of lighting's effect on function, orientation, mood, and behavior, accompanied by recommended adjustments to lighting to promote function and safety. The rationale for the need for warmer room temperatures is provided. The effects of various colors are discussed to challenge nurses to consider the therapeutic use of colors in the elderly's environment. Floor covering selection is reviewed with attention to the problems associated with carpeting. Specific characteristics of furniture that make it appealing, functional, and comfortable are described.

Because of the profound effect of sensory impairments on the health, safety, and well-being of the elderly, environmental inclusions that stimulate the senses are reviewed. Such factors include the use of various textured objects, plants, pets, music, and aromatherapy.

The physiological and emotional effects of noise are discussed. Emphasis is given to the competition of environmental noises with sounds the elderly want or need to hear in their environments.

The bathroom as a site of many accidental injuries is highlighted. Advice is provided regarding lighting, floor surfaces, faucets, tub and shower stalls, toilets, and assistive devices that can promote function and safety.

The chapter concludes with a discussion of the psychosocial considerations of the environment, including the importance of privacy, individuality, and the quality of human interactions.

The nursing diagnosis Impaired Home Maintenance Management is highlighted in this chapter.

■ Significant Displays, Tables, and Figures

Environmental Needs Based on Maslow's Hierarchy (Table 15-1)
Environmental Assessment (Table 15-2)
Examples of Therapeutic Uses of Essential Oils (Display 15-1)
Noise Levels (Display 15-2)

STUDENT OBJECTIVES

After reading this chapter, the student should be able to:

1. Discuss the significance of the environment to physical and psychosocial health and well-being.

2. List the impact of age-related changes on the function and safety of the environment.

3. Describe adjustments that can be made to the environment to promote the safety and function of older persons.

4. Identify bathroom hazards and ways to minimize them.

5. Discuss the impact of environment on psychosocial health.

■ Classroom Teaching-Learning Activities

1. Ask the students to visit at least three public places (e.g., restaurant, mall, office building) and identify features of each environment that make it either user-friendly or difficult for older adults.

2. Discuss modifications that could be made in the average hospital to make it more functional and safe for older patients.

3. Ask the students to discuss and sketch (or develop a model) for an ideal apartment for an older adult.

4. Observe and discuss the behaviors of people in environments that show different characteristics of lighting, noise, traffic flow, etc. (e.g., environments that are loud vs. quiet, busy vs. private, brightly lit vs. dim).

■ Guidelines for Evaluating Critical Thinking Exercises

1. Persons cannot focus on psychosocial and spiritual concerns if their basic physicological needs are not met.

2.
   - replace fluorescent lighting with several sources of soft lighting
   - use sheer curtains to filter sunlight
   - chairs with armrests
   - nonslip floor and tub surfaces
   - wall outlets accessible without bending

3.

- bedroom: greens, blues, soft lighting
- recreation room: yellow, bright (although nonglare), plants, pets, variety of shapes and textures
- dining room: orange and earth tones, soft lighting, contrasting colored plates and placemats

4.

- liquids on floor, harsh bright lighting, electrical appliances, poisonous substances that can be ingested accidentally, slippery tub/shower stall, hard surfaces of sink, tub, and commode

5.

- plants
- pets
- art on walls
- scents (coffee, baked goods, aromatherapy)
- use of variety of colors, textures, shapes

■ Test Questions

1. Using Maslow's framework in relation to considering environmental needs, you would expect that an older adult would:
   a. prefer surroundings that offer intellectual stimulation
   b. only be concerned with basic safety, security, and cleanliness of his or her surroundings
   c. **want to control roaches in his or her home before considering refurnishing the decor**
   d. have little interest in the mundane maintenance and housekeeping aspects of his or her home

2. An ideal room temperature for an older adult would range between:
   a. 55° and 60° F
   b. 65° and 69° F
   c. **75° and 79° F**
   d. 85° and 89° F

3. You are asked to evaluate lighting plans for a new senior citizen center. The plan that is best for an older population would be:

   a. **several diffuse sources of light along the perimeter of the room**

   b. large fluorescent lights on the ceilings at 10-foot intervals

   c. spotlights shining from the corners of the room toward the center

   d. a large bright ceiling light and several table lamps with low-watt bulbs

4. Which is least conducive to creating a therapeutic environment for an older nursing home resident?

   a. **decorating the resident's room similarly to all other residents' rooms**

   b. modifying the room to accommodate the resident's disabilities

   c. including the resident's personal possessions in the room

   d. respecting the resident's privacy and personal space

5. An example of the microenvironment is:

   a. weather

   b. traffic

   c. **furnishings**

   d. pollution

6. Which of the following soft colored lights can be useful at night in bedrooms of the elderly?

   a. blue

   b. yellow

   c. black

   d. **red**

7. True or false: Older adults can feel cold in room temperatures that feel comfortable or even warm to younger persons.

   a. **true**

   b. false

8. Describe three problems that can be caused by carpeting in the environment of older adults.

   Static cling and electricity, difficult wheelchair mobility, odor retaining, difficult to clean, can attract insects

9. Which of the following scents in the environment can have a calming effect?

    a. peppermint

    b. eucalyptus

    c. ammonia

    d. lavender

10. True or false: Entering an area 5 to 10 feet from the client is an invasion of personal space.

    a. true

    b. false

CHAPTER 16

Sexuality and Intimacy

This chapter presents issues pertaining to the older adult as a sexual being. It begins by reviewing attitudinal changes that society has experienced about sexuality, showing that the topic of sex has gone from being a taboo subject to one that is widely and openly discussed. A parallel is made in examining the development of attitudes about sex and the aged, with acknowledgment that the accepting, nonjudgmental attitude about sex in general has not been applied in the same manner to sex and the elderly. The student is encouraged to view nurses as having a part in changing attitudes by educating, counseling, and setting a good example themselves.

Differences between sexuality and sexual acts are discussed. Examples are given of ways that the elderly's sexuality is disrespected in routine caregiving activities.

Age-related differences in the sexual response cycle are outlined. Emphasis is given to the fact that adults do not lose the ability or interest in sex with age.

Major causes of sexual dysfunction among the elderly are reviewed and include the unavailability of a partner, psychological factors, physical obstacles, the effects of drugs, and cognitive impairment. Specific measures that nurses can employ to promote sexuality and intimacy in older adults are discussed with inclusion of considerations for the institutionalized elderly.

The nursing diagnosis Sexual Dysfunction is highlighted.

■ Significant Displays, Tables, and Figures

STUDENT OBJECTIVES

After reading this chapter, the student should be able to:

1. Discuss the impact of society's attitudes on the sexuality of older adults.
2. Describe sexuality.
3. List the effects of aging on sexual function.
4. List effects of reduced estrogen levels.
5. Discuss natural and pharmacologic measures to manage symptoms of menopause.
6. Describe factors that can contribute to sexual dysfunction.
7. Identify measures to promote sexuality and intimacy in the elderly.

■ Classroom Teaching-Learning Activities

1. Discuss the changes that have appeared in television and movie scripts in the portrayal of the elderly as sexual beings. Discuss stereotypes that continue to exist.
2. List barriers to sexuality and sexual function to elderly in:
   a. nursing home settings
   b. acute hospital settings
   c. private residences in the community
3. Survey common drugs used by a sample of older adults and review them for possible effects that the drug can have on sexual function. Discuss measures to compensate or assist older adults in managing these effects.
4. Ask a group of older adults to list their three major concerns and/or questions regarding their sexual function. Discuss findings.
5. Outline the content of a teaching plan on the topic of sexuality and aging for use with middle-aged and senior adults. Implement if possible.

■ Guidelines for Evaluating Critical Thinking Exercises

1.
   • people uncomfortable discussing issue
   • research fairly recent
   • myths regarding elders being uninterested and incapable
   • ageism

2.

- sexuality entails identity as male or female
- physical sex act concerned with orgasm, physical stimulation

3.

- maintain good health
- correct health conditions
- assist with promoting good appearance
- respect sexual identity and role

4. Refer to Table 16-2

5. Refer to Table 16-1

6.

- negative effect: not assessing sexual function, failing to counsel as to effects of disease and drugs on sexual function, not respecting privacy during caregiving, not assisting with grooming and dressing, belittling elders who display sexual interest
- positive effect: opposite of factors listed under negative effect

■ Test Questions

1. Mrs. James is a 77-year-old resident of a senior housing complex in which you are working. You observe that she attends social functions with excessive amounts of makeup as compared with other women in her group. Your best action is to:

   a. ask her the reason for her need to use excessive amounts of cosmetics

   b. privately inform her that her cosmetics use is inappropriate

   c. observe her for other signs of alterations in judgment

   d. do nothing if she is satisfied with her appearance

2. You are listening to a group of senior citizens discuss changes in their sexual function. Which of the following statements would you know to reflect an abnormality?

   a. "Sometimes my vagina is so dry my husband can't enter me without causing me discomfort."

   b. "I have been unable to achieve an orgasm since I had my hysterectomy years ago."

   c. "It takes longer for my penis to become fully erect when I prepare to have intercourse."

   d. "My ejaculations are not as strong and forceful as they were when I was younger."

3. A happily married couple in their forties tells you that they enjoy intimacy and hope their sex life can continue as they age. Your best response is:

   a. "Even when sexual activity diminishes, you'll continue to share your love."

   b. "You are unusual to be sexually active at your age now, so you also may be unusual in your sexual activity when you reach old age."

   c. "Continuing the relationship you now share as you age should help you to enjoy sex into your late life."

   d. "Any problems you hear older adults express about sexual function are due to psychological rather than real physical causes."

4. List three age-related factors that can negatively affect sexuality in late life.

   Ageism, chronic diseases, lack of partner, reduced vaginal secretions

5. True or false: Sexuality includes the expression and perception of oneself as a man or woman.

   a. true

   b. false

6. Which is an expected age-related change in the sexual response cycle?

   a. increased intensity of orgasm

   b. shorter period for erection to be achieved

   c. lack of full erection

   d. reduced sex flush

7. Describe the impact of the following conditions on sexual function:

   prostatitis   alcoholism

   prolapsed uterus   Refer to Table 16-2

   diabetes mellitus

8. List five drugs that can affect sexual function and the type of problem they can create.

9. Hormonal replacement therapy is known to do all of the following except:

   a. reduce symptoms of menopause

   b. decrease risk of heart disease

   c. prevent osteoporosis

   d. elevate low-density lipoprotein (LDH) cholesterol levels

10. True or false: Older men can maintain an erection for a longer period before ejaculation than can younger men.

    a. true

    b. false

Safe Medication Use

Chapter 17 highlights challenges to the older individual's safe and therapeutic use of drugs. Although the elderly represent approximately 12% of the population, they consume nearly one-third of all prescription drugs and numerous over-the-counter medications. The volume of drugs consumed and their potential interactions, along with the impact of age-related changes, result in significant risk for adverse reactions in the elderly. This chapter reviews these issues and offers recommendations for safe drug use.

Major drug groups used by the elderly are discussed in relation to principles and risks, interactions, and related nursing guidelines.

■ Significant Displays, Tables, and Figures

Risk Factors for Medication Errors (Display 17-1)
Teaching Tool: Tips for Safe Drug Use (Display 17-2)
Alternative and Complementary Therapies as Substitutes for Drugs (Display 17-3)
Interactions Among Popular Drug Groups (Table 17-1)
Examples of Food and Drug Interactions (Table 17-2)
Potential Adverse Effects of Selected Herbs (Table 17-3)

STUDENT OBJECTIVES

After reading this chapter, the student should be able to:

1. Describe the unique aspects of pharmacokinetics and pharmacodynamics in the aged.
2. List measures to promote safe drug use.
3. Discuss alternatives to medications.

■ Classroom Teaching-Learning Activities

1. Discuss risks associated with the elderly's self-administration of drugs and measures to reduce these risks.

2. Survey a group of senior citizens for their knowledge about their medications (e.g., intended use, side effects, interactions). Discuss findings.

3. Review popular magazines and newspapers read by the older population for the publications' advertisements by drug companies. Discuss the effects of this marketing on older consumers and their attitudes about medication use.

■ Guidelines for Evaluating Critical Thinking Exercises

1. Age-related changes: decreased intracellular fluid, increased gastric pH, decreased gastric blood flow and motility, reduced cardiac output and circulation, slower metabolism, proportionate increase in adipose tissue, reduced renal filtration rate

2. Refer to Display 17-2

3.
   - prefilled drug containers
   - charting system
   - buddy system for someone to check on administration

4. Refer to Display 17-3; discuss options

■ Test Questions

1. The drugs most commonly prescribed for the elderly are:
   a. **cardiovascular agents**
   b. laxatives
   c. psychotropic drugs
   d. antidepressants

2. The absorption, distribution, metabolism, and excretion of drugs is referred to as:
   a. pharmacodynamics
   b. **pharmacokinetics**
   c. synergism
   d. biological life

3. True or false: Dehydration can result in higher plasma drug levels.
   a. **true**
   b. false

4. Describe three nonpharmacological measures to reduce hypertension that could be attempted before antihypertensive therapy is initiated.

   Meditation, yoga, progressive relaxation, hawthorn berry supplement, dietary modification

5. You note that an 80-year-old client who is taking digoxin has headache, nausea, dizziness, and diarrhea and refuses food. Her pulse rate, usually in the range of 76 to 84 beats, is 60. You notify the physician, who tells you to advise the client to take an antidiarrheal medication and an analgesic. The physician also tells you to observe the symptoms. You question the physician about the possibility of digitalis toxicity. The physician tells you this is not a problem because the serum drug level taken yesterday was within normal limits. Your best action would be to:

   a. follow the physician's instructions

   b. withhold the digoxin

   c. omit all medications for a 24-hour period and note the client's symptoms closely

   d. question the possibility of digitalis toxicity being present despite the normal drug level in the blood

6. An anticoagulant can interact with all of the following except an:

   a. antidiabetic drug

   b. anti-anxiety drug

   c. anti-depressant

   d. anti-hypertensive

7. True or false: A client who is consuming 12 or more aspirin tablets can experience a vitamin C deficiency.

   a. true

   b. false

8. True or false: An older adult's consumption of several protein-bound drugs concurrently can cause increased effects of the drugs.

   a. true

   b. false

9. True or false: Biological half-life of drugs can be reduced in older adults.

   a. true

   b. false

10. Describe three measures nurses can use with older adults to enhance the benefits of drug therapy.

    Maintain good hydration; promote activity; be familiar with and avoid drug–drug, drug–herb, and drug–food interactions; use guided imagery

CHAPTER 18

Immunity and Infectious Diseases

The final chapter in this unit describes unique factors related to the immune system in late life and the problems these can create. A variety of age-related changes increase the body's susceptibility to infections and diminish the strength of the immune response. For this reason, gerontological nurses need to help elders strengthen their immune systems and take precautions against infections.

Common infections are reviewed, including urinary tract infections, prostatitis, influenza, pneumonia, tuberculosis, vaginitis, herpes zoster, and scabies. Display 18-3 offers a discussion of control of a scabies outbreak in a long-term care facility.

Measures to promote immunologic health are discussed, such as diet, exercise, immunization, stress management, mind–body interventions, and careful use of antibiotics.

■ Significant Displays, Tables, and Figures

Major Components of the Immune System (Display 18-1)
The Severity of Pneumonia Increases with Age (Display 18-2)
Control of a Scabies Outbreak in a Long-Term Care Facility (Display 18-3)
Examples of Adverse Effects from Antibiotics (Display 18-4)

STUDENT OBJECTIVES

After reading this chapter, the student should be able to:

1. List major changes in immunologic function as a result of aging.

2. Describe unique features of the common infections of older adults.

3. Discuss natural approaches to boosting immunologic health.

4. Describe the risks associated with overuse and misuse of antibiotics.

■ Classroom Teaching-Learning Activities

1. Discuss factors other than age-related physical changes that contribute to elders' high risk of infections.

2. Review the health records of several patients to determine:

   a. whether they have a history of an infection

   b. symptoms that indicated they had infections

   c. measures used to prevent and manage infections other than antibiotics

3. Discuss reasons for Americans' past high reliance on antibiotics and reasons that this attitude now is changing.

■ Guidelines for Evaluating Critical Thinking Exercises

1.
   - good nutrition, daily vitamin/mineral supplement
   - regular exercise
   - immunizations
   - stress management
   - importance of assertiveness, trust, continued psychological growth
   - careful use of antibiotics

2. Younger generations are exposed to more pollutants, eat more processed foods, live more stressful lifestyles than previous generations

3.
   - people wanted "quick fixes" to health problems rather than slower but more natural approaches
   - until recent years preventive care was not emphasized; focus was on treating problems rather than preventing them
   - marketing of drugs
   - lack of knowledge of negative effects from overusing antibiotics

4.
   - medications used as first lines of defense to treat infections rather than utilizing measures to increase body's natural ability to resist and fight infection
   - this can be changed by instructing patients in measures to enhance immunity, advising them about risks of antibiotic misuse

■ Test Questions

1. True or false: Although the elderly have a reduced antibody response to pneumococcus, influenza, and tetanus vaccines, these vaccines are recommended.

   a. true

   b. false

2. Once the body has been exposed to _____, it stores information about it in the immune system's memory.

   a. an antibody

   b. a T-cell

   c. an antigen

   d. a B cell

3. The most common infection of the elderly is:

   a. pneumonia

   b. influenza

   c. prostatitis

   d. urinary tract infection

4. True or false: Most urinary tract infections in women are due to *Escherichia coli.*

   a. true

   b. false

5. Temperatures of 99° F or higher may not occur with infections in older adults because:

   a. infections cause temperature decreases in the elderly

   b. depressed immune responses in the elderly interfere with normal responses to infection

   c. baseline temperatures can be lower than normal in the elderly; thus, elevations do not appear as high

   d. all of the above

6. True or false: Not only has cranberry juice been found to be ineffective in preventing urinary tract infections, but it also has been shown to promote the growth of bacteria in the bladder.

   a. true

   b. false

7. Which of the following could be contraindications for administering an influenza vaccine?

   a. history of Guillain-Barré syndrome

   b. egg allergy

   c. febrile condition

   d. all of the above

8. True or false: Tuberculosis in the elderly is usually the result of a reactivation of an earlier TB infection.

   a. true

   b. false

9. Scabies is caused by:

   a. a mite

   b. a virus

   c. a blood-borne pathogen

   d. any of the above

10. True or false: Studies have identified personality traits such as assertiveness, ability to trust, and sense of control over one's life to be consistent with strong immune systems.

    a. true

    b. false

UNIT III

Common
Geriatric Conditions

This section focuses on health problems that are common among the elderly. Most chapters are organized by the system that is primarily involved, such as cardiovascular conditions, musculoskeletal conditions, and neurological conditions. A separate chapter is dedicated to sensory deficits due to the scope of these conditions. The chapters on health conditions of specific systems are organized similarly in that they present a discussion of measures to facilitate health, review major diagnoses and care measures specific to the diagnoses, offer general nursing measures, describe complementary therapies that could prove useful, and list resources to assist in increasing knowledge and caregiving skills related to specific conditions.

Chapter 28 reviews conditions related to mood and cognition. Measures to promote mental health are discussed, as well as unique challenges faced in old age that affect mental health. Of the major disorders reviewed, particular attention is paid to delirium, dementia, and depression. As with the other chapters in this section, nursing measures, including complementary therapies, and resources are provided.

The intent of this section is to acquaint the student with the unique features of diseases in the older population and to encourage him or her to balance illness and disability with wellness and capability so that the older adult will be empowered for maximum independence and self-care.

CHAPTER 19

Cardiovascular Conditions

Chapter 19 begins with a discussion of measures to facilitate cardiovascular health. Particular emphasis is given to the role of nutrition, exercise, effective stress management, and the avoidance of cigarette smoking.

Display 19-3 describes factors to consider during the assessment that can aid in detecting cardiovascular problems and determining the impact of these conditions on the individual. To trigger the student's thinking, Table 19-1 lists nursing diagnoses that may be present in persons with cardiovascular problems. A sample care plan for the patient with congestive heart failure is offered in Display 19-4.

The unique features of cardiovascular disease are presented; the conditions reviewed are congestive heart failure, pulmonary heart disease, coronary artery disease, hypertension, arrhythmias, bacterial endocarditis, rheumatic heart disease, and syphilitic heart disease.

Peripheral vascular diseases are discussed in this chapter. Conditions reviewed include arteriosclerosis, special problems of the diabetic patient, aneurysms, varicose veins, and venous thromboembolism. Features and treatment of these conditions are highlighted.

Ischemic foot lesions and loss of a limb are special problems addressed in the discussion of general nursing interventions. The role of complementary therapies such as yoga, acupressure, and herbs is included to stimulate the student's thinking in the direction of natural and noninvasive measures to manage peripheral vascular conditions.

In addition to the specific measures included in the discussion of individual diagnoses, general nursing considerations are described for persons with cardiovascular disease; these include keeping the patient informed, preventing complications, promoting normality, and using complementary therapies. Resources for persons with various cardiovascular conditions are listed for the student to explore for further information and patient information literature.

■ Significant Displays, Tables, and Figures

Nursing Diagnoses Related to Cardiovascular Conditions (Table 19-1)
Dietary Guidelines for Reducing the Risk of Cardiovascular Disease (Display 19-1)
Nutritional Supplements for Cardiovascular Health (Display 19-2)
Assessment of the Cardiovascular System (Display 19-3)
Sample Care Plan for the Patient with Congestive Heart Failure (Display 19-4)

STUDENT OBJECTIVES

After reading this chapter, the student should be able to:

1. List measures that promote cardiovascular health.

2. Identify unique features of common cardiovascular diseases in the elderly.

3. Describe nursing actions to assist patients with cardiovascular conditions.

■ Classroom Teaching-Learning Activities

1. Review the content of a health education program for teaching senior citizens ways to promote cardiovascular health. If possible, have the students implement this teaching plan.

2. Discuss the challenges in effecting a change in lifestyle practices to promote cardiovascular health in older adults.

3. Obtain a speaker or video to teach the students about alternative health practices (e.g., yoga, meditation) that can promote cardiovascular health and help cardiovascular disease.

4. Identify various support groups in the community to assist persons who have cardiovascular disease.

■ Guidelines for Evaluating Critical Thinking Exercises

1.
   * jobs and lifestyles require less physical activity
   * high stress levels
   * high consumption of fats

2. Discuss impact on physical, emotional, and social well-being.

3.
   * diet
   * activity (schedule when activity can be increased)
   * medications
   * sexual activity
   * symptom recognition
   * stress management

4.

- eat low-fat, high-fiber diet
- limit consumption of alcohol
- regularly engage in physical exercise
- avoid smoking and exposure to cigarette smoke
- effectively manage stress
- establish loving relationships

■ Test Questions

1. A reduction in the following dietary product can aid in reducing cardiovascular disease:

   a. highly processed food

   b. monounsaturated oils

   c. complex carbohydrates

   d. fiber

2. Nitrates can cause dizziness after their administration due to:

   a. flushing effect

   b. hypotensive effects

   c. tachycardia

   d. pooling of blood in pulmonary vessels

3. You observe a nursing assistant caring for an older patient who is recovering from an MI. The nursing assistant tells the patient that she will soon be allowed to walk, should call the nursing assistant to request assistance to use the commode rather than a bedpan for toileting, should use the overhead trapeze to lift and reposition herself, and will use an armchair when sitting out of bed. Of the comments made to the patient, the one you see as needing correcting is that the patient:

   a. will soon be allowed to ambulate

   b. should use a commode rather than a bedpan

   c. should lift and reposition herself with an overhead trapeze

   d. will use an armchair when sitting out of bed

4. An older patient with hypertension asks you why it seems that nearly all her friends have this condition. Your best response is:

   a. "Most people say they have hypertension while they really do not."

   b. "Hypertension is normal in late life."

c. "Physicians misdiagnose hypertension to a greater degree than other conditions."

d. **"Hypertension increases in incidence with age and is the most common heart disease in late life."**

5. Which of the following group of symptoms is least likely to be associated with congestive heart failure?

a. bilateral ankle edema, agitation, dyspnea

b. **capillary fragility, shortness of breath, orthopnea**

c. confusion, weight gain, shortness of breath

d. wandering at night, moist crackles, ankle edema

6. Potential complications of myocardial infarction in older adults that the nurse should observe include:

a. elevating blood pressure and flushing

b. esophageal pain and weight loss

c. increased anterior-posterior chest diameter and depression

d. **edema and decreasing blood pressure**

7. True or false: For older persons with mild hypertension, meditation can be more advisable than antihypertensive drugs.

a. **true**

b. false

8. True or false: When significant edema is present in an older adult, excessive activity should be avoided because it can increase the circulation of toxic wastes and cause intoxication.

a. **true**

b. false

9. Which of the following treatment orders for a patient with ischemic foot lesions would you question as being unusual?

a. a systemic antibiotic

b. chemical debridement of eschar

c. **a topical antibiotic**

d. range-of-motion exercises

10. Which of the following measures can be useful in preventing vagal stimulation?

a. **preventing constipation**

b. providing a soft diet

c. massaging the extremeties

d. reducing edema

CHAPTER 20

Respiratory Conditions

This chapter begins with a discussion of the impact of aging on respiratory health. Age-related changes often enable respiratory problems to easily develop and to be more difficult to manage than in younger age groups. These changes also can cause an atypical presentation of symptoms, as is exemplified when pneumonia presents with altered cognition rather than chest pain in some elders.

Specific suggestions for facilitating respiratory health are offered, including promoting activity, avoiding cigarette smoke, effectively managing respiratory illness, using drugs safely so as not to mask symptoms of respiratory illness, and controlling environmental pollutants. The student is encouraged to include measures to facilitate respiratory health into the care plan of all elders.

General measures to consider in assessing respiratory health are outlined in Display 20-1. The unique signs and symptoms and treatment measures for selected respiratory disorders are reviewed; included in this review are asthma, chronic bronchitis, emphysema, lung cancer, and lung abscess. Nursing measures to reduce the risk of complications are discussed, such as maintenance and promotion of oral health, close observation, and techniques to remove secretions. Unique risks in the use of oxygen with older adults are described. Herbs, acupressure, and yoga are among the complementary therapies discussed that can offer benefit to some patients with respiratory conditions.

A sample care plan for the patient with emphysema is offered in Display 20-2. Resources to assist patients with various respiratory conditions are listed at the end of the chapter.

■ Significant Displays, Tables, and Figures

Cautious Use of Oxygen (Figure 20-1)
Assessment of Respiratory Conditions (Display 20-1)
Sample Care Plan for the Patient with Emphysema (Display 20-2)

STUDENT OBJECTIVES

After reading this chapter, the student should be able to:

1. List the impact of age-related changes on respiratory health.

2. Describe measures to facilitate respiratory health in the elderly.

3. Discuss the risks, symptoms, and care considerations associated with selected respiratory illnesses.

4. List interventions that can aid in preventing complications and promoting self-care in older persons with respiratory conditions.

■ Classroom Teaching-Learning Activities

1. Ask the students to design and, if possible, implement a breathing exercise program to teach to older adults.

2. List environmental and personal health care practices that have changed in the past 20 years that could positively or negatively affect respiratory health.

3. Survey the community for the various smoking cessation programs that exist and discuss the advantages and disadvantages of each program.

■ Guidelines for Evaluating Critical Thinking Exercises

1.
   • cigarette smoking
   • air pollution
   • inactivity
   • poor infection-control practices

2.
   • infections can develop more easily
   • altered symptomatology can delay recognition and diagnosis
   • older adults experience higher rates of morbidity and mortality

3.
   • smoking cessation
   • breathing exercises
   • importance of physical activity
   • infection-control practices
   • good dietary practices
   • value of pneumococcal and influenza vaccines

4. Refer to Figure 20-1.

■ Test Questions

1. Age-related changes can affect respiratory health in all of the following ways except:

   a. mucus plugs develop easily

   b. pain sensations can be altered

   c. less air remains in the lungs after exhalation

   d. the risk of aspiration is greater

2. Which condition would you expect to be associated with a blue or gray discoloration of the upper extremity?

   a. emphysema

   b. chronic bronchitis

   c. lung abscess

   d. all of the above

3. True or false: A lung abscess can result from tuberculosis, lung cancer, or aspiration of foreign material.

   a. true

   b. false

4. It is recommended that oxygen be administered at lower levels to an older person with COPD because:

   a. oxygen cannot be fully absorbed by the diseased alveoli

   b. nonproductive coughing can be stimulated by high oxygen levels

   c. carbon dioxide can accumulate with high oxygen administration levels

   d. a dependency on the mechanical provision of oxygen can result from chronic administration of high levels

5. True or false: Age-related changes in the mucous membranes can result in excess mucus production and an increased risk of infection.

   a. true

   b. false

6. True or false: Deep breathing exercises that focus on forced expirations are contraindicated for older clients who have respiratory conditions.

   a. true

   b. false

7. True or false: Older adults with emphysema should be advised against receiving influenza and pneumococcal vaccines.

   a. true

   b. false

8. Overuse of sympathomimetic bronchodilating nebulizers by older asthmatics can result in:

   a. cardiac arrhythmias

   b. pneumonia

   c. pulmonary edema

   d. esophageal ulceration

9. Seventy-eight-year-old Mr. Clark states that he was prescribed cromolyn sulfate for control of his asthma and although he has taken the drug for several days, he has not seen any improvement. Your best response is to:

   a. advise him that several weeks of therapy may be necessary for benefits to be realized

   b. explain that this drug will help to prevent infections but does not impact symptoms

   c. suggest that he discontinue the drug

   d. explain that this drug was not prescribed for his asthma

10. True or false: Nonproductive coughing is equally advantageous to the older client as productive coughing and should be promoted.

   a. true

   b. false

CHAPTER 21

Gastrointestinal Conditions

This chapter reviews factors that affect gastrointestinal health and some of the disorders commonly affecting this system in late life. The point is made that although gastrointestinal problems are not as life threatening as other systems' problems, these disorders can create many concerns for the elderly and can have an impact on the quality of life. Factors to consider in assessing gastrointestinal problems are described in Display 21-1.

The disorders discussed include anorexia, dry mouth, dental problems, esophageal diverticulum, hiatal hernia, cancer of the esophagus, peptic ulcer, cancer of the stomach, diverticulosis, diverticulitis, cancer of the colon, acute appendicitis, chronic constipation, fecal impaction, fecal incontinence, cancer of the pancreas, and biliary tract disease. Unique characteristics of these conditions in the elderly are reviewed. Sample care plans for patients with hiatal hernia and altered bowel eliminaiton are offered in Displays 21-2 and 21-3.

Points to remember in gavage feedings are described in the nursing considerations section. Resources to assist patients with gastrointestinal problems are listed at the end of the chapter.

■ Significant Displays, Tables, and Figures

STUDENT OBJECTIVES

After reading this chapter, the student should be able to:

1. List factors to consider when assessing gastrointestinal problems.

2. Discuss the unique features of gastrointestinal disorders in late life, including anorexia, dry mouth, dental problems, esophageal diverticulum, hiatal hernia, cancer of the esophagus, peptic ulcer, cancer of the stomach, diverticulosis, diverticulitis, cancer of the colon, acute appendicitis, chronic constipation, fecal impaction, fecal incontinence, cancer of the pancreas, and biliary tract disease.

3. Describe measures to assure safe nasogastric feedings.

■ Classroom Teaching-Learning Activities

1. Ask the students to survey a group of senior citizens about their oral hygiene practices. Based on findings, direct the students to design an educational program to promote oral health.

2. Discuss factors that have a positive or negative influence on appetite of the elderly.

3. List the risks to health of chronic use of antacids and laxatives.

■ Guidelines for Evaluating Critical Thinking Exercises

1.
   - weight loss
   - fatigue, lack of energy to engage in ADLs
   - change in appearance, poor body image and self-concept
   - potential for altered cognition, depression

2.
   - emphasis on preventive dentistry
   - correcting dental problems and saving teeth versus pulling them
   - abolishing myth that tooth loss is normal part of aging

3. Exercise, high-fiber foods, plenty of liquids, establishing regular time for bowel elimination

4. Discuss physical, cognitive, emotional, and social risks to GI health and nutritional status and measures to reduce these risks.

■ Test Questions

1. Your patient with hiatal hernia describes his practices for managing this condition. Of the following practices, the one you would recommend changing is:

   a. eating a small snack prior to retiring for the night

   b. eliminating spicy foods and carbonated beverages from the diet

   c. sleeping with the head of the bed slightly elevated

   d. eating five small-portioned meals throughout the day

2. Your 83-year-old patient has a poor appetite and distended abdomen. She complains of abdominal discomfort and small amounts of diarrhea. You notice fecal matter on her nightgown. Your best action is to consult with the physician regarding the need for:

   a. an antidiarrheal medication

   b. a digital rectal exam

   c. lower GI studies

   d. stool cultures

3. Which older person is at greatest risk for esophageal cancer?

   a. an Asian woman with high fiber intake

   b. a black woman with uncontrolled diabetes

   c. a black man who is alcoholic

   d. a white man with a history of antacid use

4. True or false: A reduction in saliva can increase the risk of oral cavity infections.

   a. true

   b. false

5. A particularly high risk to the older client with esophageal diverticulum is:

   a. wasting syndrome

   b. malabsorption syndrome

   c. gastritis

   d. aspiration

6. True or false: The geriatric patient with a peptic ulcer who is using an antacid can experience an alteration in bowel elimination.

   a. true

   b. false

7. The type of diet that is most likely to contribute to diverticulosis is:

   a. low-fiber, low-residue

   b. high-fiber, high-residue

   c. high-calorie, high-residue

   d. high-sodium, high-glucose

8. True or false: Fecal occult blood testing is not as effective for the early detection of colonic tumors in the aged as it is for younger adults.

   a. true

   b. false

9. List three nursing measures to prevent constipation in older clients.

   Encourage high-fiber diet, offer fluids, suggest/assist with physical activity, identify foods that stimulate bowel elimination for the individual client (prunes, bananas, etc.)

10. Who of the following is the most likely person to develop gallstones?

    a. a 45-year-old woman

    b. a 70-year-old woman

    c. a 50-year-old man

    d. an 80-year-old man

CHAPTER **22**

Musculoskeletal Conditions

Chapter 22 reviews the prevention and management of common musculoskeletal problems in late life. The role of diet and activity in promoting good musculoskeletal function is discussed. Display 22-1 highlights assessment of musculoskeletal problems with an emphasis on not only identifying the presence of these conditions, but also exploring the impact these problems have on the older adult's function and general status.

Selected disorders are reviewed, including fractures, osteoarthritis, rheumatoid arthritis, osteoporosis, and gout. Measures to prevent and manage falls are described.

Because of the high prevalence of arthritis among the elderly, a sample care plan for the patient with osteoarthritis is provided.

Pain management receives special attention under the General Nursing Measures section. Backrubs, positioning, diversional activities, acupuncture, and chiropractic therapy are among the pain management measures discussed. Display 22-3 presents guided imagery as a method of pain management and offers a sample script that could be used. The importance of preventing injury and promoting independence is described.

■ Significant Displays, Tables, and Figures

Gait Disturbances (Table 22-1)

Good Sources of Calcium (Table 22-2)

Nursing Diagnoses Related to Musculoskeletal Problems (Table 22-3)

Assessment of Musculoskeletal Problems (Display 22-1)

Sample Care Plan for the Patient with Osteoarthritis (Display 22-2)

Guided Imagery for Pain Management (Display 22-3)

Risk Factors for Osteoporosis (Display 22-4)

Correct Method for Stepping (Figure 22-2)

Normal Versus Osteoporotic Bone Tissue (Figure 22-3)

Methods for Reducing Musculoskeletal Pain (Figure 22-4)

Self-Care Devices to Help the Patient Achieve the Maximum Independence Possible (Figures 22-5, 22-6, 22-7)

STUDENT OBJECTIVES

After reading this chapter, the student should be able to:

1. List measures to facilitate musculoskeletal function.

2. Describe the unique characteristics and management of fractures, osteoarthritis, rheumatoid arthritis, osteoporosis, and gout.

3. List measures that can be used for managing musculoskeletal pain.

4. Describe nursing measures to prevent injury and promote independence of the elderly who have musculoskeletal problems.

■ Classroom Teaching-Learning Activities

1. Discuss factors that may positively and negatively affect musculoskeletal function for future generations of elderly.

2. Ask the students to design a pain management patient education program that utilizes measures other than medications.

3. Ask the students to survey popular media for advertisements for arthritic pain relief and discuss the approaches they find.

■ Guidelines for Evaluating Critical Thinking Exercises

1.
   - busy schedules
   - often feel physical effects more than when younger
   - less opportunity

2.
   - safe clothing and shoes
   - proper stepping off curb
   - how to fall safely
   - good calcium intake
   - using good judgment

3.

   Pain, limited mobility, effects of medications can interfere with psychological well-being and decrease socialization

4.

- massage
- therapeutic touch
- guided imagery
- heat
- homeopathic remedies
- acupuncture

5.

- unfamiliar environment
- effects of medications (sedation, dizziness, confusion)
- hospital bed
- equipment and clutter

6. Explore community resources (e.g., Arthritis Foundation, pain management clinics, osteoporosis support groups)

■ Test Questions

1. All of the following are true about fractures in the elderly except:

   a. compression fractures of the vertebrae are the most common type

   b. the bones of the elderly are more brittle than those of the young and break easily

   c. a fracture may not be apparent on the first x-ray

   d. fractures heal at a slower rate in the elderly

2. The musculoskeletal problem that is the leading cause of physical disability in the aged is:

   a. osteoporosis

   b. osteoarthritis

   c. rheumatoid arthritis

   d. fractured femur

3. A patient tells you that he is taking colchicine for his "joint problem." You know that this drug is used in the treatment of:

   a. osteoporosis

   b. osteoarthritis

   c. rheumatoid arthritis

   d. gout

4. You would expect that a patient with multiple sclerosis would have which type of gait?

    a. ataxic

    b. foot-slapping

    c. spastic

    d. scissors

5. Which is not an accurate description of osteoarthritis?

    a. Osteoarthritis affects weight-bearing joints most frequently.

    b. Osteoarthritis typically affects one joint rather than several.

    c. Wear and tear of the joints has a role in the development of osteoarthritis.

    d. Osteoarthritis does not cause the systemic symptoms as does rheumatoid arthritis.

6. True or false: Most cases of rheumatoid arthritis develop after age 65.

    a. true

    b. false

7. Which of the following conditions is least likely to be responsible for the development of osteoporosis?

    a. Parkinson's disease

    b. reduction in production of estrogens and androgens

    c. long-term heparin therapy

    d. prolonged immobility

8. True or false: Osteoporosis can be responsible for a reduction in height of older adults.

    a. true

    b. false

9. Crepitation and Heberden's nodes are associated with:

    a. gout

    b. rheumatoid arthritis

    c. osteoarthritis

    d. osteoporosis

10. List three measures that can assist persons with osteoarthritis.

    Heat application, massage, mild exercise of joints, yoga, swimming

CHAPTER 23

Genitourinary Conditions

This chapter reviews what are sometimes difficult disorders for the elderly to discuss: genitourinary problems. Display 23-1 outlines factors to review in the assessment of genitourinary conditions that can help them to be identified. General measures to promote healthy function of this system are discussed and include good fluid intake, activity, and regular prostate and gynecologic examinations.

The discussion of urinary incontinence explains the various types of incontinence and offers specific measures for promoting continence. Display 23-2 lists factors for the nurse to consider in assessing the incontinent patient, and Display 23-3 offers a sample care plan for the incontinent patient.

Other conditions reviewed include bladder cancer, renal calculi, glomerulonephritis, pyelonephritis, infections and tumors of the vulva, cancer of the vagina, cancer of the cervix, perineal herniation, dyspareunia, breast cancer, benign prostatic hypertrophy, and prostate cancer.

The importance of treating patients who have these problems with dignity is reinforced. Resources to assist patients with genitourinary problems are listed at the end of the chapter.

■ Significant Displays, Tables, and Figures

Assessment of the Genitourinary System (Display 23-1)
Factors to Review When Assessing the Incontinent Patient (Display 23-2)
Sample Care Plan for the Patient with Incontinence (Display 23-3)
The Patient Recovering from Prostate Surgery (Display 23-4)
Nursing Diagnoses Associated with Genitourinary Problems (Table 23-1)
Measures to Facilitate Voiding (Figure 23-1)

STUDENT OBJECTIVES

After reading this chapter, the student should be able to:

1. List measures to promote genitourinary health.

2. Describe the various types of urinary incontinence and measures to aid them.

3. Discuss the characteristics and treatment of selected genitourinary problems.

■ Classroom Teaching-Learning Activities

1. Ask the students to list factors in the hospital, nursing home, and community setting that could promote functional incontinence and recommendations for preventing or controlling them.

2. Design a patient education program for older women that teaches them self-examination of breasts.

3. Discuss the psychosocial implications of incontinence.

■ Guidelines for Evaluating Critical Thinking Exercises

1. Refer to Display 23-2

2.
   - general: have cause of incontinence identified
   - stress: Kegel exercises, biofeedback, medications
   - urge: Kegel exercises, toileting schedule, biofeedback, medications
   - overflow: toileting schedule, Credé's method, intermittent catheterization, medications
   - functional: provide assistance, bedside commode

3.
   - misconceptions regarding sexual function in late life: teach, counsel, clarify
   - medications that decrease libido and sexual function: instruct on impact of medications, discuss with patient and physician possibility of trying nonpharmacologic means to manage condition
   - disability or symptoms of patient or partner: advise in positions, medication schedules, and assistive measures that can facilitate sexual function, refer to support groups

4. Older adults may not have been instructed in self-exams; often, emphasis is toward younger adults. Assess patient's knowledge of self-exam and instruct as necessary.

5.
   - assist patient in obtaining evaluation and correction of problem, if possible
   - assist patient in using effective incontinence brief, condom catheter
   - do not discuss incontinence in presence of others

6. Identify local support groups, chapters of the American Cancer Society, and other resources.

■ Test Questions

1. Mr. Clark has an enlarged prostate gland that has caused irritation of the bladder and led to incontinence. This type of incontinence is:

   a. **urgency**

   b. stress

   c. functional

   d. neurogenic

2. Which is not a true statement about benign prostatic hypertrophy?

   a. A majority of older men have some degree of benign prostatic hypertrophy.

   b. Treatment of benign prostatic hypertrophy can include prostatic massage.

   c. Transurethral surgery is the most common prostatectomy approach used.

   d. **Symptoms of benign prostatic hypertrophy appear abruptly.**

3. A risk factor that can promote bladder cancer is:

   a. carbonated beverages

   b. **cigarette smoking**

   c. multiple pregnancies

   d. prolonged immobility

4. If a postvoid residual is ordered for a patient, one would expect that:

   a. the patient will be asked to void within 15 minutes after the first void

   b. **the patient will be catheterized within 15 minutes after voiding**

   c. a midstream urine sample will be obtained and sent to the lab

   d. a record will be maintained to determine the length of time between voiding

5. True or false: The test for prostate-specific antigen (PSA) is 100% reliable in detecting prostate cancers in older men.

   a. true

   b. **false**

6. True or false: Functional incontinence can be improved with surgery or medications.

   a. true

   b. **false**

7. True or false: Urinary tract infections come in second only to pneumonia as the leading infections of the aged.

   a. true

   b. false

8. Which symptom is least likely to be associated with glomerulonephritis?

   a. elevated blood pressure

   b. hypothermia

   c. edema

   d. anorexia

9. True or false: Most older women who are sexually active can be expected to develop senile vaginitis as a chronic problem.

   a. true

   b. false

10. Describe the reason that older women are at high risk for burns from a douche.

   Decreased ability to discriminate various temperatures and sense pain

Neurologic Conditions

Chapter 24 reviews disorders of the neurologic system. The point is made that this system's status impacts every aspect of activities of daily living. Although many neurologic conditions are not preventable, the reduction of risk factors can prevent or minimize some conditions; these risk factors include cigarette smoking, obesity, ineffective stress management, elevated cholesterol, hypertension, and head trauma.

The selected conditions that are reviewed include Parkinson's disease, transient ischemic attack, and cerebrovascular accident. Display 24-3 offers a care plan for the patient who has had a cerebrovascular accident.

The discussion of general nursing measures focuses on the importance of promoting independence and preventing injury. Resources to assist patients with neurologic problems are listed at the end of the chapter.

■ Significant Displays, Tables, and Figures

Assessment of Neurological Function (Display 24-1)
Nursing Diagnoses Related to Neurological Function (Table 24-1)
Examples of Subtle Indications of Neurological Problems (Display 24-2)
Sample Care Plan for the Patient Convalescing from a Cerebrovascular Accident (Display 24-3)

STUDENT OBJECTIVES

After reading this chapter, the student should be able to:

1. List measures to reduce the risk of neurological problems.

2. Outline factors to consider in assessing neurological conditions.

3. Describe the features and treatment of Parkinson's disease, transient ischemic attacks, and cerebrovascular accidents.

■ Classroom Teaching-Learning Activities

1. Discuss the care of the patient with a stroke from the acute through the rehabilitative phases.

2. Demonstrate and describe assistive devices to promote the independence of persons with neurological conditions. Invite a rehabilitation specialist to speak to the students, if possible.

■ Guidelines for Evaluating Critical Thinking Exercises

1.
- avoid abuse of alcohol and other substances
- do not smoke
- protect head when bicycling or engaging in other activities in which head injury is a risk
- maintain vital signs within normal range
- prevent falls
- use seat belts when driving

2. Refer to Display 24-3

3.
- factors that worsen symptoms: tension, frustration
- offer psychological support, patience; avoid rushing

4. Explore community resources for local chapters of stroke and Parkinson's disease associations.

■ Test Questions

1. A drop attack would cause a patient to have:
   a. muscular flaccidity in the legs but no loss of consciousness
   b. muscular flaccidity in the legs with a loss of consciousness
   c. residual weakness and paralysis
   d. rapid declines in cognition

2. Which sign is least likely to be associated with Parkinson's disease?
   a. increased tremor with purposeful movements
   b. muscle rigidity
   c. monotone voice
   d. drooling

3. During the neurological assessment, you note that the nurse asks the patient to repeat the sounds "la, la, la." The nurse is doing this to assess the function of the:

   a. facial nerve

   b. lips

   c. tongue

   d. pharynx

4. An abnormal finding during the neurological assessment is:

   a. blinking of eye when cornea is touched

   b. ability to rapidly tap finger on a table surface

   c. flexion of toes when sole of foot is stroked

   d. calling a watch a clock

5. List three factors that can aid in preventing some neurological problems.

   • avoid abuse of alcohol and other substances

   • do not smoke

   • protect head when bicycling or engaging in other activities in which head injury is a risk

   • maintain vital signs within normal range

   • prevent falls

   • use seat belts when driving

6. True or false: Signs associated with transient ischemic attack seldom last for more than a few minutes and can vary depending on the location of the area of the brain involved.

   a. true

   b. false

7. List five conditions that increase the risk for cerebrovascular accident.

   • hypertension

   • arteriosclerosis

   • diabetes

   • gout

   • anemia

   • hypothyroidism

   • myocardial infarction

   • dehydration

   • history of TIA

   • cigarette smoking

8. True or false: Personality changes experienced by persons with neurological conditions are more likely related to approaches by caregivers than the conditions themselves.

    a. true

    b. false

9. Which is not necessary in the care of a person who has had a cerebrovascular accident?

    a. talking to the person during caregiving activities

    b. speaking in a louder voice

    c. devising an easy means of communication

    d. providing consistency of caregivers and routines

10. True or false: Anticholinergic drugs can exacerbate glaucoma.

    a. true

    b. false

Sensory Deficits

Chapter 25 presents the significance of good sensory function to health, safety, and well-being. A variety of factors can affect sensory status, such as aging and disease processes. Sensory deficits can compound other problems that the elderly possess. Display 25-1 guides the student through the assessment of the senses.

General measures to facilitate optimal sensory function are described. These include regular ophthalmological examinations, prompt evaluation of symptoms, and protection from trauma.

The signs and management of visual deficits are presented. Cataracts, glaucoma, macular degeneration, detached retina, and corneal ulcers are highlighted. Display 25-3 offers a care plan for the patient with open-angle glaucoma. Hints for compensating for visual deficits are provided in Figure 25-1.

A discussion of hearing deficits and related nursing interventions is included. Practical tips for communicating with persons who have hearing deficits are provided, along with a display and figure that discuss hearing aids.

Other sensory deficits are reviewed, along with suggestions for compensating for them. The importance of touch is emphasized. Resources to assist people with visual and hearing impairments are listed at the end of the chapter.

■ Significant Displays, Tables, and Figures

Assessment of Sensory Function (Display 25-1)
Nursing Diagnoses Associated with Sensory Deficits (Table 25-1)
Nutrients Beneficial to Vision (Display 25-2)
Administering Eye Medications Using Tear Duct Occlusion Technique (Display 25-3)
The Patient with Open-Angle Glaucoma (Display 25-4)
Correcting Cerumen Impaction (Display 25-5)
Living with a Hearing Aid (Display 27-6)
Compensating for Visual Deficits in the Aged (Figure 25-1)
Measuring Intraocular Pressure by Use of a Tonometer (Figure 25-2)
Problems Affecting the Ears of Aged People (Figure 25-3)
Types of Hearing Aids (Figure 25-4)

STUDENT OBJECTIVES

After reading this chapter, the student should be able to:

1. Discuss the impact of sensory deficits on health, safety, and well-being.

2. List measures to facilitate optimal sensory function.

3. Describe the signs and management of cataracts, glaucoma, macular degeneration, detached retina, and corneal ulcers.

4. Describe hearing deficits common in the elderly and related nursing interventions.

5. Outline factors to consider in assessing sensory function.

6. Describe the types and care of hearing aids.

■ Classroom Teaching-Learning Activities

1. Guide the students through a sensory deprivation simulation experience. Pair the students, with one being the "patient" and the other the caregiver/observer. Have the patients create sensory deficits by stuffing their ears with cotton, blindfolding themselves or wearing eyeglasses that have been smeared with petroleum jelly, wearing gloves, and stuffing their nose. Instruct their partners to perform various activities, such as feeding, ambulating, etc. Instruct some of the caregivers/observers to restrain their patients in wheelchairs and leave them unattended for several minutes. Discuss feelings and time perceptions of the patients and observations of the caregivers/observers.

■ Guidelines for Evaluating Critical Thinking Exercises

1.
   - obtain annual vision and hearing evaluations
   - avoid exposure to loud noises, bright sunlight
   - have infections and other conditions treated promptly

2. Symptoms of glaucoma are subtle and gradual.

3. Refer to Display 25-4.

4. Refer to Figure 25-1.

5. Consult with an occupational therapist, a hearing specialist, or medical supply companies regarding assistive devices available.

6. Explore community resources for local chapters of American Council for Blind, Hearing and Speech Society, etc.

■ Test Questions

1. Your patient complains of "itching ears," and upon inspection you note a buildup of cerumen in the ear canal. Your best action is to:

   a. loosen the cerumen with a cotton-tipped applicator

   b. remove the cerumen with use of tweezers

   c. irrigate the ear canal

   d. do nothing and allow the cerumen to drain naturally

2. Which of the following set of symptoms is consistent with acute glaucoma?

   a. flashes of light, feeling of coating over the eye, blurred vision

   b. loss of central vision, tired eyes, tearing

   c. loss of peripheral vision, tired eyes, halos around lights

   d. blurred vision, severe eye pain, nausea

3. Mrs. Connor, 78 years old, is a new participant in the adult day care program. She shows you her medications, which include pilocarpine hydrochloride; she tells you this is for her "eye problem." Which eye disorder would the drug most likely be used for?

   a. open-angle glaucoma

   b. diabetic retinopathy

   c. cataracts

   d. macular degeneration

4. All of the following can have a negative impact on Mrs. Connor's eye disorder except:

   a. strenuous exercise

   b. lying perfectly flat

   c. aggressive coughing

   d. emotional stress

5. A new ophthalmology clinic is opening, and you have been asked to tour it and offer suggestions regarding its appropriateness for older adults. You notice that signs are printed in large black letters, the color scheme uses cheerful bright colors, the interviewer's desk backs against a large window to allow the patient to view the outdoors, and the doorways are a contrasting color from the walls. A suggestion you could make to enhance the elderly's function in the environment would be to:

   a. use low tone rather than bright colors

   b. print signs with blue letters against a green background

   c. cover the window with a sheer curtain or tinted glass

   d. paint the doorways the same color as the walls

6. True or false: All people develop some degree of lens opacity as they age.

   a. true

   b. false

7. Which of the following symptoms is not likely to be associated with cataracts?

   a. eye pain

   b. blurred vision

   c. sensitivity to glare

   d. loss of vision

8. You are told that your aged patient has macular degeneration. You would expect this patient to display:

   a. reduced peripheral vision

   b. loss of central vision

   c. eye pain

   d. night blindness

9. List three conditions that can cause hearing impairments.

   Exposure to loud noises, recurrent ear infections, ototoxic drugs, diabetes, tumors

10. Which is not an expected experience while using a hearing aid?

   a. amplification of environmental noises

   b. distortion of speech

   c. constant buzzing or ringing

   d. ease of reverberation

CHAPTER 26

Dermatologic Conditions

C hapter 26 reviews common disorders of the most visible system of the body. Benign and malignant skin problems significantly increase with age, and suggestions are offered to reduce their occurrence. There is a discussion of cosmetic surgery and the nurse's role in counseling and educating patients who seek this option.

Display 26-1 reviews factors to consider in assessing skin status. Specific guidelines for staging pressure ulcers are provided in Display 26-3.

Selected dermatologic disorders are reviewed with a discussion of their signs and treatment. The disorders featured include pruritus, keratoses, seborrheic keratoses, malignant melanoma, stasis dermatitis, and pressure ulcers.

The importance of promoting normalcy is discussed under general nursing considerations. The various alternative therapies that could be used to naturally treat skin problems are described.

■ Significant Displays, Tables, and Figures

Assessment of Skin Status (Display 26-1)
Techniques Used to Treat Pressure Ulcers (Display 26-2)
Stages of Pressure Ulcers (Display 26-3)
Common Location for Pressure Sores (Figure 26-1)
Nursing Diagnoses Related to Dermatological Problems (Table 26-1)

STUDENT OBJECTIVES

After reading this chapter, the student should be able to:

1. Describe measures to facilitate healthy skin status.

2. List the characteristics and treatment of pruritus, keratoses, seborrheic keratoses, malignant melanoma, and stasis dermatitis.

3. Describe prevention, treatment, and staging of pressure ulcers.

4. Discuss alternative therapies that can be used in the treatment of skin problems.

■ Classroom Teaching-Learning Activities

1. Identify several immobile older patients. Assign students to check the patients' pressure points at 2-hour, 1½-hour, 1-hour, and ½-hour intervals and identify the length of time various patients could remain in the same position before showing signs of redness. Discuss findings and implications for individualized turning schedules.

2. Ask the students to survey several older adults for the presence of skin problems and discuss their findings.

3. Invite a cosmetic surgeon to discuss cosmetic surgery options available to help aging people look more youthful. Discuss views on cosmetic surgery and list the issues nurses should address with older adults who are exploring cosmetic surgery.

■ Guidelines for Evaluating Critical Thinking Exercises

1.

   • pressure ulcers: convey dependent state, diminish independence, may necessitate institutional care

   • malignant melanoma: may trigger grief, depression, anger; others may disengage

2. Check patient's pressure points for redness after being in same position for half hour; if no signs of pressure, allow patient to remain in position for 1 hour and check pressure points again; if no pressure apparent, continue increasing time intervals for as long as 2 hours. Patient should be turned at intervals before redness is shown.

3.

   • benefits: may improve body image and self-concept, fosters acceptance in youth-oriented society, assists in maintaining competitiveness in labor force

   • risks: complications from surgery; disappointment with results; expectations may not be realized, leading to depression

4. Brainstorm on items that could be included in protocol.

■ Test Questions

1. You read on a patient's health record that she has a stasis ulcer on her right ankle. You could reasonably expect her leg to look:

    a. pale with purple streaks running along the posterior

    b. smooth, shiny, and swollen

    c. pigmented, cracked, and exudative

    d. purulent, smooth, moist

2. The nurse who has taken care of 80-year-old Mrs. Howard reports to you that Mrs. Howard needs to be turned at least hourly. You could accurately believe that:

    a. the nurse is being overly cautious and that q2h turning will be sufficient

    b. Mrs. Howard develops signs of pressure if in the same position longer than 1 hour

    c. an hourly turning schedule could tax the energy of Mrs. Howard

    d. this turn schedule is more for psychosocial rather than physical benefit

3. Which is the largest lesion?

    a. macule

    b. papule

    c. nodule

    d. tumor

4. Dark, wart-like projections on the skin surface that are not accompanied by swelling or redness are:

    a. seborrheic keratosis

    b. malignant melanoma

    c. keratosis

    d. eschar

5. A pressure ulcer that presents as a blister or shallow crater is a:

    a. stage 1

    b. stage 2

    c. stage 3

    d. stage 4

6. The most common dermatologic problem among the elderly is:
   a. stasis ulcer
   b. pressure ulcer
   c. malignant melanoma
   d. pruritus

7. Which individual is at highest risk for developing malignant melanoma?
   a. an 85-year-old African-American woman
   b. a 25-year-old man with dark skin
   c. a 72-year-old woman with fair skin
   d. a 75-year-old man with an olive complexion

8. True or false: Eschar on a pressure ulcer should not be removed until granulation is present.
   a. true
   b. false

9. True or false: The incidence of malignant melanoma increases with age.
   a. true
   b. false

10. List three ways of preventing shearing forces.
    Don't elevate bed more than 30 degrees, don't allow patients to slide in bed, lift instead of pulling patients when moving them

Metabolic and Endocrine Conditions

The endocrine system enables the body to grow and develop, maintain homeostasis, and respond to stress and injury. The complexities of this system are discussed in Chapter 27.

Diabetes, the seventh leading cause of death in the elderly, is presented. Differences in assessing diabetes in the elderly are reviewed, including the need to use age-adjusted gradients for evaluating glucose tolerance test results.

Self-care requirements for managing diabetes and the special challenges this presents for older adults are discussed. Factors reviewed include the ability of the older adult to handle a syringe and vial, self-testing for blood glucose, exercise, diet, and medications.

Older diabetics are at high risk for many complications; those reviewed in this chapter include hypoglycemia, hyperglycemia, peripheral vascular disease, retinopathy, drug interactions, cognitive impairments, and neuropathies.

Because education is important to patient compliance with the diabetes management program, the student is offered a sample content for diabetic patient education in Display 27-1 and guidelines for patient education in Display 27-2. Care plan guidelines are featured, also.

Additional conditions that are reviewed include hypothyroidism, hyperthyroidism, and hyperlipidemia. Resources to assist patients with metabolic and endocrine conditions are listed at the end of the chapter.

■ Significant Displays, Tables, and Figures

STUDENT OBJECTIVES

After reading this chapter, the student should be able to:

1. Describe age-related differences in the diagnosis, presentation, and management of diabetes mellitus.

2. Outline a teaching plan for the older person with diabetes.

3. List self-care requirements of the older diabetic.

4. Identify common complications of the older diabetic.

5. Describe signs of hypothyroidism, hyperthyroidism, and hyperlipidemia.

■ Classroom Teaching-Learning Activities

1. Review the laboratory blood results for a group of older adults and discuss findings related to blood glucose.

2. Discuss challenges faced by older adults who are newly diagnosed with diabetes.

3. Discuss unique problems that can be encountered in teaching older adults.

4. List interactions that hypoglycemic agents can have with other drugs that are commonly used by the elderly.

■ Guidelines for Evaluating Critical Thinking Exercises

1. Age-adjusted gradients using higher levels of blood glucose are used to evaluate the test.

2.
   - complications can develop that can threaten independence, well-being, and life

3.
   - urinary frequency, weight changes, fatigue may be associated with normal aging rather than the disease

4.
   - low-fat diet
   - herbal supplements (e.g., garlic)
   - exercise, yoga, tai chi
   - stress management

■ Test Questions

1. Symptoms related to hypoglycemia in the elderly include all of the following except:

   a. elevated blood pressure

   b. confusion

   c. glaucoma

   d. impotence

2. True or false: Diet and lifestyle modifications are of minimum benefit to older adults with hyperlipidemia; therefore, medications are the primary treatment.

   a. true

   b. false

3. In interviewing your patient with diabetes, you learn that he plans to join a fitness center and begin a training program. An accurate statement to him would be:

   a. "You may need to increase your food intake to compensate for your extra energy expenditure."

   b. "You may need to have your insulin dosage readjusted because your exercise could cause your insulin to absorb more quickly."

   c. "You may need to reduce your insulin because you will be producing more glucose in your body."

   d. "You will probably need to add an oral hypoglycemic agent to your insulin to cover the increase in glucose that you will experience."

4. Which of the following symptoms is not typically associated with hypothyroidism?

   a. diarrhea

   b. depression

   c. dry skin

   d. anorexia

5. True or false: A glucose level that would be abnormal for a young adult could fall within the normal range for an older individual.

   a. true

   b. false

6. Insulin requirements can be reduced by a diet:
   a. high in simple carbohydrates
   b. low in fiber
   c. high in fat
   d. high in complex carbohydrates

7. True or false: Tachycardia, restlessness, and perspiration may not be present in the older diabetic with hypoglycemia.
   a. true
   b. false

8. List three complications of diabetes that the older adult can experience.
   Peripheral vascular disease, retinopathy, cognitive impairment, coronary artery disease, neuropathies

9. True or false: Hyperthyroidism is more prevalent in older adults than hypothyroidism.
   a. true
   b. false

10. True or false: Diabetes ranks as the third leading cause of death of persons over age 85 years.
    a. true
    b. false

Conditions Affecting Mood and Cognition

Issues pertaining to mental health and illness are presented in Chapter 28. The chapter begins with emphasis on the emotional strengths of the elderly, gained through a lifetime of challenges from situations unknown to most individuals of younger generations. The realities of cognitive function are discussed, and Display 29-1 outlines the many considerations in assessing mental status in the elderly.

The promotion of mental health in older adults is discussed. Good mental health practices throughout the lifetime, remaining engaged in activities, feeling secure and valued, and maintaining physical health are among the components of good mental health that are reviewed.

Of the mental illnesses reviewed, major attention is given to delirium, dementia, and depression as the leading disorders. The student is urged to differentiate signs of delirium from those of dementia to ensure appropriate treatment for the patient. Practical caregiving measures are offered, as in a case study featuring the care of a patient with Alzheimer's disease. Other mental health issues reviewed in this chapter include suicide, anxiety, alcohol abuse, paranoia, and hypochondriasis. Displays offer specific information on recognizing alcohol abuse, causes of confusion, drugs that can cause depression, and the management of common behavioral problems.

Nurses play an important role in caring for the elderly with mental health problems. Interventions reviewed include monitoring medications, promoting a positive self-concept, and managing behavioral problems.

■ Significant Displays, Tables, and Figures

Assessment of Mental Health (Display 28-1)
Potential Causes of Impaired Cognition (Display 28-2)
Sundowner Syndrome (Display 28-3)
Case Study (Display 28-4)
Drugs Than Can Cause Depression (Display 28-5)
Antidepressants (Display 28-6)
Basic Goals in Caring for Depressed Patients (Display 28-7)
Possible Indications of Alcohol Abuse (Display 29-8)
Criteria for Diagnosing Alcoholism (Display 28-9)
Nursing Diagnoses Related to Mental Health Problems (Table 28-1)

Checklist for Documenting Drugs and Behavior (Table 28-2)
Understanding and Managing Common Behavioral Problems (Table 28-3)
Stages of Alzheimer's Disease (Figure 28-1)

STUDENT OBJECTIVES

After reading this chapter, the student should be able to:

1. Discuss the emotional strength possessed by the elderly as a result of their life experiences.

2. List measures to promote mental health in the elderly.

3. Describe the characteristics and care of delirium, dementia, depression, anxiety, alcohol abuse, paranoia, and hypochondriasis.

4. Discuss general nursing interventions to care for mental illnesses and behavioral problems.

■ Classroom Teaching-Learning Activities

1. Discuss the needs of the community-based Alzheimer's victim and special problems faced by family caregivers. Ask the students to locate resources in the community to help persons with Alzheimer's disease and their caregivers.

2. List and discuss factors that contribute to delirium in older adults.

3. Ask the students to review the health records of several patients who are diagnosed as having Alzheimer's disease and to determine whether adequate evaluations were performed to rule out other possible causes of dementia.

4. Discuss reasons for alcoholism being overlooked in some older adults.

■ Criteria for Evaluating Critical Thinking Exercises

1. Factors considered could include ageism, purposelessness, pressure to conform with youthful appearance, alcohol and drug abuse.

2.
   - unfamiliar environment
   - drug reactions
   - hypoxia
   - hemorrhage
   - hypothermia, fever
   - infection
   - pain

3. Discuss role changes, caregiver responsibilities, financial burdens.

4. Both have altered cognition; patient may not be properly assessed.

5.
   - older drinkers tend not to be "loud drunks"
   - symptoms can be easily mistaken for "growing old" or health conditions (e.g., fatigue, confusion, inattention to self-care, neglect of home maintenance)

6. Refer to Display 28-1.

7.
   - hearing and vision impairments
   - real risk of being victimized

■ Test Questions

1. To assist a patient who is experiencing sundowner syndrome, you could:
   a. keep the room completely dark at night and bright during the day
   b. restrict fluids and activity in the evening
   c. avoid contact and interruptions with the patient
   d. keep some form of lighting in the room at night

2. For the person with Alzheimer's disease, suicide risk is greatest:
   a. early in the disease's course
   b. in the late stage of the disease
   c. when physical deterioration occurs
   d. there is not a significant risk of suicide at any stage

3. The most frequent problem psychiatrists treat in the elderly is:
   a. Alzheimer's disease
   b. delirium
   c. depression
   d. paranoia

4. Which disorder can the symptoms of depression mimic?
   a. dementia
   b. delirium
   c. anxiety
   d. hypochondriasis

5. Which is an inaccurate statement regarding alcoholism in the elderly?

    a. A majority of older alcoholics have been chronic alcohol abusers.

    b. Higher levels of alcohol are necessary to intoxicate older people.

    c. Older alcoholics recover more slowly than do younger alcoholics.

    d. Polyneuropathy and cardiac disorders can result from alcoholism.

6. True or false: Less than 5% of suicides are committed by persons age 65 and older.

    a. true

    b. false

For questions 7 to 10, explain the differences between delirium and dementia in reference to:

7. causes

    delirium: anything that disrupts body's homeostasis

    dementia: destruction of brain tissue

8. onset of symptoms

    delirium: rapid

    dementia: gradual, subtle

9. treatment

    delirium: correct underlying cause

    dementia: slow deterioration through medications, behavioral interventions, provide assistance with ADLs

10. prognosis

    delirium: reversible and good if underlying cause treated in timely manner

    dementia: irreversible, progressive decline

UNIT IV

Gerontological Care Issues

The reality that a majority of older adults are affected by at least one chronic illness supports the need for Chapter 29, Living in Harmony With Chronic Conditions. After a discussion of the scope and challenges of chronic illness, the chapter presents practical considerations in helping older adults to live with chronic conditions. Healing versus curing is discussed to sensitize the student to the importance of promoting a high quality of life in which the elderly learn to live with, not for, their illnesses. Unique chronic care goals and care guidelines are offered.

Chapter 30 presents Rehabilitative Care. The challenges of living with a disability are discussed. Principles of rehabilitative nursing that can be applied to general gerontological nursing practice are reviewed. Specific guidelines for assessing functional status are offered. Special rehabilitative measures that commonly are used in gerontological care are described and include range-of-motion exercise, use of mobility aids, bowel and bladder training, and maintaining and promoting mental function.

Acute Conditions is the topic of Chapter 31. Although many health care professionals who work in acute care settings do not consider themselves providers of geriatric care, about one-half of all hospital beds are filled by persons over age 65 and one-quarter of all inpatient hospital days are used by persons over age 75 years. Unique aspects of surgical care of older patients are described. Emergency conditions and related nursing measures are reviewed, as are measures to prevent and manage infections. The nurse's role in effective discharge planning is discussed.

Geriatric Nursing in Long-Term Care Facilities is the focus of Chapter 32. The development of long-term institutional care is traced to aid students in gaining a perspective for some of the current problems of nursing in this setting. Standards and nursing responsibilities in nursing facilities are discussed. Students are challenged to envision a new paradigm for long-term care facilities that shifts from a biomedical to a holistic, healing model.

With greater numbers of families providing hands-on care for elderly relatives, the topic of Chapter 33, Family Caregiving, was added to this edition. Various family structures and roles are reviewed. The dynamics of family relationships are addressed, including parent–child relationships, grandparenting, and marriage. The scope of family caregiving and needs of the caregiver are discussed. The topic of elder abuse is included in this chapter as it relates to being associated with caregiver stress. Consideration is given to the positive aspects of caring for an elder relative.

Chapter 34 addresses the commonly faced issues in gerontological care of Death and Dying. Coping mechanisms used by dying individuals are outlined with related nursing interventions. The support required not only of the dying individual but also of family, friends, and caregiving staff are discussed.

Chapter 35 reviews the important concern of Legal Aspects of Gerontological Nursing. The protection of the elderly's legal rights is an important function of the gerontological nurse due to the vulnerability and multiple health, social, and economic challenges the elderly face. Furthermore, the unique staffing profile of some geriatric care settings (e.g., the low ratio of professional to nonprofessional staff in nursing homes), regulatory requirements, and the issue of liability reinforce the need to build legal safeguards into gerontological practice. Malpractice, consent, competency, supervision, drugs, restraints, telephone orders, no-code orders, advance directives, and abuse are the specific legal risks discussed.

The Ethics of Caring is the focus of Chapter 36. Some of the changes that increase ethical dilemmas for nurses are discussed. Philosophies guiding ethical thinking and the ethical principles of beneficence, nonmaleficence, justice, fidelity, and autonomy are described. Guidance is offered for making ethical decisions.

The many settings for gerontological nursing practice are surveyed in Chapter 37, The Continuum of Services. Students are acquainted with the wide range of services available to elders and challenged to consider the use of traditional services.

Challenges of the Future, Chapter 38, closes the book with a review of future issues the gerontological nurse faces, including advocating research, educating caregivers, developing new roles, balancing priorities, and promoting holistic practices.

CHAPTER 29

Living in Harmony With Chronic Conditions

This chapter highlights the frequently encountered issue of chronic illness in the older population and the challenges of living with chronic conditions. The chapter begins with the facts about the prevalence of chronic illnesses in the elderly. The difference between healing and curing is discussed, with suggestions offered for stimulating patients' self-healing capabilities; the intent is to promote the important role of nurse as healer and to empower patients as active participants in their care.

Chronic care goals are presented, which include maintaining or improving self-care capacity, managing the disease effectively, boosting the body's healing abilities, preventing complications, delaying deterioration and decline, achieving the highest possible quality of life, and dying with comfort and dignity. These goals are contrasted to the acute care goals of diagnosing, treating, and curing.

Factors to consider in assessing and planning for chronic care needs are discussed. Specific recommendations are given for maximizing care activities, which include appropriately selecting a physician, using a coach, increasing knowledge, using resources, making smart lifestyle decisions, and using alternative therapies to enhance conventional treatments. Issues to consider as the nurse evaluates the long-term effectiveness of the care of chronically ill elders are discussed.

■ Significant Displays, Tables, and Figures

Major Chronic Conditions of Older Adults (Display 29-1)
Potential Nursing Diagnoses Associated with Ten Major Chronic Problems of the Elderly (Table 29-1)
Chronic Care Goals (Display 29-2)
Functions of a Chronic Care Coach (Display 29-3)
Steps in Chronic Care Coaching (Display 29-4)
Alternative Therapies for Chronically Ill People (Display 29-5)

STUDENT OBJECTIVES

After reading this chapter, the student should be able to:

1. Discuss the scope of chronic illness among the elderly population.
2. Differentiate healing versus curing.
3. List chronic care goals.
4. Outline components of assessment of chronic care needs.
5. Discuss approaches to maximize the benefits of conventional treatments.
6. Identify alternative therapies that could benefit chronically ill persons.

■ Classroom Teaching-Learning Activities

1. Design patient education programs for patients with the following conditions:

   a. COPD

   b. arthritis

   c. hypertension

   d. dementia

   Identify community resources to assist caregivers and to assist patients affected with these conditions. Also, review alternative therapies that could be used to assist these patients.

2. Discuss factors that cause health care professionals to show less interest in chronic than in acute care issues.

3. Discuss how the current health care practices and lifestyle of persons ages 25 to 45 years will affect their development and management of chronic conditions as they age.

■ Criteria for Evaluating Critical Thinking Exercises

1. Encourage students to share their personal reactions.

2. Discuss possible nursing actions related to nursing diagnoses that could be identified, e.g.:

   • Activity intolerance

   • Anxiety

   • Ineffective individual coping

   • Noncompliance

   • Disturbance in self-concept

   • Sexual dysfunction

3.
- have not been taught in nursing or medical schools
- attitudes that anything outside biomedical system is not valid
- cultural insensitivity
- lack of familiarity with research validating

4.
- provide knowledge
- offer several options for treatment
- utilize complementary therapies

5. Encourage discussion of how students see an elder's life affected by arthritis, heart disease, vision and hearing impairments, respiratory conditions, diabetes, etc.

■ Test Questions

1. The major chronic condition of the elderly is:
    a. diabetes mellitus
    b. hypertension
    c. dementia
    d. arthritis

2. All of the following are chronic care goals except:
    a. improving self-care capacity
    b. eliminating the disease
    c. preventing complications
    d. dying with comfort and dignity

3. A 70-year-old patient has been dependent on oxygen for his chronic respiratory condition for several years and is unable to leave his home without becoming severely fatigued and short of breath. You are aware that he has been taught about his illness and has demonstrated competency in self-care activities. On a recent home visit he told you that he once hiked into the Grand Canyon and plans to do so again next year with his grandson upon the grandson's graduation from college. You could interpret this to mean that this patient:
    a. may be in need of psychological support
    b. may be in need of additional education
    c. is going to cure himself from his illness
    d. will most likely be able to meet this challenge

4. You are working with a family who is providing care in the home for a relative with Alzheimer's disease. The family made a commitment to this relative years ago that they "would never put her in a nursing home." You note that the family is suffering considerable economic and social hardships in caring for this relative and that some members are experiencing physical effects from the lack of sleep and direct care demands of the relative. Your best action is to:

   a. wait until they ask for help

   b. initiate a referral for nursing home placement and inform them afterwards that you have determined this to be the best action

   c. meet with the family and introduce the topic of adult day care or nursing home care

   d. give them positive feedback for their caregiving and allow them to keep their commitment

5. True or false: A majority of the elderly have a chronic condition.

   a. true

   b. false

6. List three measures that nurses can use to boost the body's healing abilities.

   Good nutrition, stress management, exercise, herbs (e.g., echinacea, ginseng, garlic), positive attitude, use of humor

7. The primary purpose of a chronic care coach is to:

   a. provide support, assistance, and feedback

   b. provide direct care

   c. confront the client when there is noncompliance

   d. coordinate the efforts of the interdisciplinary team

8. List three factors that can change the patient's ability to manage an illness.

   Change in physical status, impaired cognition, depression, reduced income, loss of caregiver/support system

9. True or false: In chronic care nursing, the nurse's primary concern is the welfare of the patient regardless of the impact on the family.

   a. true

   b. false

10. Explain what is meant by the statement *Successes in chronic care are measured differently from those in acute care.*

   Cure and improvement may not be possible in chronic care; maintaining patient at current status or delaying deterioration can indicate success in chronic care.

CHAPTER 30

Rehabilitative Care

This chapter reviews the aspects of care that promote optimal function in persons with various impairments. The impact of a disability is discussed in terms of losses and challenges to daily life. Due to the scope of disabling conditions in the older population, rehabilitation is suggested as an integral part of gerontological nursing. Principles that could guide the gerontological nurse in rehabilitative care are described.

Guidelines are offered for assessing functional capacities. Table 30-1 lists specific actions that could cause patients to be evaluated as totally independent, partially independent, or dependent in each of the ADLs.

Some of the major considerations in rehabilitative care are reviewed, such as proper positioning, range-of-motion exercises, use of mobility aids, and bowel and bladder function. The student is encouraged to view the maintenance and promotion of mental function as important to rehabilitation.

Organizations that can be important resources in rehabilitative efforts are listed at the end of the chapter.

■ Significant Displays, Tables, and Figures

Disability, Impairment, Handicap (Display 30-1)
Terms Used to Describe Joint Mobility (Display 30-2)
Care Plan for Altered Urinary Elimination Pattern: Incontinence (Display 30-3)
Care Plan for Altered Bowel Elimination: Incontinence (Display 30-4)
Assessing Capacity to Perform Activities of Daily Living (Table 30-1)
Tool for Assessing Range of Motion (Table 30-2)
Proper Alignment in Various Positions (Figure 30-1)
Range-of-Motion Exercises (Figure 30-2)
Proper Use of Mobility Aids (Figure 30-3)

STUDENT OBJECTIVES

After reading this chapter, the student should be able to:

1. Discuss challenges of living with a disability.

2. List the principles of rehabilitative nursing.

3. Describe characteristics of total independence, partial independence, and dependence.

4. Identify proper body alignment in various positions.

5. Describe range-of-motion exercises.

6. Discuss the proper use of mobility aids.

7. Describe measures that stimulate mental function.

8. Identify resources to assist persons in their rehabilitation.

■ Classroom Teaching-Learning Activities

1. Supervise the students in performing range-of-motion exercise with several patients.

2. Ask the students to demonstrate the correct use of canes, walkers, and wheelchairs.

3. Instruct the students to interview a patient with a disability to learn about the challenges he or she faces in living with the disability.

■ Guidelines for Evaluating Critical Thinking Exercises

1. An imability to perform an activity (disability) can lead to an impairment in that an abnormality is evident, and this can progress to a handicap in which a limitation in the ability to fulfill a role is present.

2. Encourage students to discuss how they would be personally affected by a disability.

3.
   - people may view the disabled person as totally incapable and not see capabilities
   - persons with physical disabilities may be treated in a patronizing manner or as though they had mental disabilities
   - people may not understand or respect the disabled person's desire and need to enjoy intimate/romantic relationships

4. Encourage students to explore local community resources.

■ Test Questions

1. Which is a valid statement regarding a patient's success in living with a disability?

   a. **Attitude and coping capacity can mean more to rehabilitative efforts than the severity of the disability.**

   b. Attitudes toward living with a disability bear little resemblance to attitudes toward other issues faced in life.

   c. Reactions toward the disability will seldom change once established.

   d. Family response toward a patient's disability has minimal effect on the patient.

2. All of the following are important to rehabilitation except:

   a. demonstrating hope and optimism

   b. preventing complications

   c. **treating all persons with similar disabilities similarly**

   d. providing time and flexibility

3. You are supporting a patient's thigh and hip as she exercises her knee and ankle. This is an example of:

   a. active exercise

   b. passive exercise

   c. **active assistive exercise**

   d. partial passive exercise

4. You are observing a patient ambulating with a cane. He has right-sided weakness and is holding the cane in his left hand. As he walks he advances the cane with his left leg and then advances his right leg. Based on this observation you would advise him to:

   a. advance his right leg before his left leg and the cane

   b. **advance the cane with his right leg**

   c. place the cane in his right hand

   d. change nothing

5. List three factors that can influence a patient's reaction to a disability.

   Previous attitudes, personality, experiences, lifestyle, reaction of significant others

6. Which finding would indicate that an exercise needed to be stopped?

   a. resting heart rate of 90; exercise heart rate of 118

   b. resting BP 110/76; exercise BP 122/84

   c. pallor

   d. flushed face

For questions 7 to 10, state whether the activity is an ADL: activity of daily living, or IADL: instrumental activity of daily living.

7. Administering medications: IADL

8. Traveling in the community: IADL

9. Preparing a meal: IADL

10. Dressing: ADL

CHAPTER 31

Acute Conditions

Acute conditions, the focus of Chapter 31, are an often underemphasized aspect of geriatric care. Older adults constitute a significant proportion of acute hospital patients; they also present special challenges in the management of acute illnesses due to their altered norms, symptomatology, and responses to treatment. This chapter discusses measures nurses can employ to reduce the risks associated with acute conditions and acute hospitalizations.

Considerations associated with surgical care are presented. Specific guidelines are given for preoperative, operative, and postoperative procedures. Emphasis is given to the prevention of complications and to the promotion of function to help the elderly achieve maximum benefit from surgical procedures.

Unique factors that cause emergency conditions to be more problematic in older adults are discussed. Principles guiding emergency care of the elderly are presented, as is a review of selected emergencies in Display 31-2.

There is a discussion of factors responsible for the high risk of infection in the elderly and measures nurses can take to prevent infections.

The chapter concludes with a review of the importance of discharge planning, particularly in the current climate of abbreviated hospital stays.

■ Significant Displays, Tables, and Figures

Nursing Diagnoses Related to Surgical Intervention (Table 31-1)
Common Complicating Conditions in Elderly Surgical Patients (Table 31-2)
Potential Risks of Older Adults during Hospitalization (Display 31-1)
Review of Selected Emergencies (Display 31-2)
Factors Contributing to the High Risk for Infection in the Elderly (Display 31-3)

STUDENT OBJECTIVES

After reading this chapter, the student should be able to:

1. List specific risks associated with surgical procedures in the elderly and ways to reduce these risks.

2. Identify major emergency conditions experienced by older adults and goals of managing these conditions.

141

3. Describe factors responsible for the high risk of infection in the elderly and general nursing measures to reduce the risk.

4. Discuss the significance of early discharge planning during hospitalization.

■ Classroom Teaching-Learning Activities

1. Ask the students to survey the ages of patients on one medical-surgical unit in an acute hospital and identify the number of patients who are over age 65 years. Have the students review the records of several of these patients and note the adjustments that have been made, or should have been made, to care as a result of age.

2. Discuss human and physical components of the acute hospital that could pose problems for elderly patients.

3. Have the students design an ideal medical-surgical unit for older patients.

■ Guidelines for Evaluating Critical Thinking Exercises

1.
- schedule that allows ample rest between activities
- prevention of pressure ulcers
- orientation
- maintenance of stable environmental temperature (approximately 75° F)
- monitoring for adverse drug effects
- cautious monitoring of oxygen therapy, IV infusions
- factors to consider in evaluating delirium

2. Risks:
- falls, injury
- pressure ulcers
- chronic incontinence
- loss of dignity and independence
- inability to return home

Plans to assist daughter:
- referral for home health care
- advice on environmental modifications and assistive devices
- instruction on safe medication use, importance of position changes, pressure ulcer prevention, diet

3.
  - maintain good health status
  - obtain influenza and pneumococcal vaccines
  - avoid crowds during flu season
  - drink plenty of fluids
  - practice good hygiene

4.
  - misconception that altered cognition, fatigue, weight loss are normal
  - misconception that surgery is too risky for elders

■ Test Questions

1. An ideal hospital room for older patients should include all of the following except:
   a. use of nightlights
   b. room temperature of 75° F
   c. bright sunlight shining through the windows
   d. control of noise

2. Which is a true statement about surgery and the elderly?
   a. Better health states of the elderly have resulted in the need for fewer surgeries for today's elderly population than in previous generations.
   b. Surgical intervention, although not responsible for adding more years to an older person's life, can increase the function of the remaining years.
   c. Prolonged surgery reduces complications in the elderly.
   d. The elderly have a smaller margin of physiological reserve than younger patients.

3. One of the major complications of the elderly intra- and post-operatively is:
   a. hypothermia
   b. hypertension
   c. hypoglycemia
   d. hypovolemia

4. The most common infection of the elderly is:
   a. pneumonia
   b. urinary tract infection
   c. septicemia
   d. furuncle

5. During the admission assessment a 76-year-old patient tells you that she has fallen several times in recent months, although she has not injured herself. You could accurately determine that:

   a. the risk of serious fall-related injury in this patient is small

   b. the patient's risk of falls will decrease with age

   c. this patient needs to be restrained during the hospitalization

   d. her risk of falling is greater than in someone who never fell

6. True or false: Most older adults are more independent and functional at discharge from a hospital than they were at admission.

   a. true

   b. false

7. True or false: Inhaled anesthesias are eliminated more slowly from the body of an older adult than from a younger person.

   a. true

   b. false

8. List three factors that contribute to the high risk of infections in the elderly.

   Refer to Display 31-3 for a listing of factors.

9. True or false: An older diabetic with an infection may experience a lack of glycemic control.

   a. true

   b. false

10. Describe three factors that the nurse should consider in planning for an older patient's discharge from a hospital.

    Self-care capacity, availability of caregivers, prognosis, health insurance

CHAPTER 32

Nursing in Long-Term Care Facilities

This chapter traces the development of long-term care from early models of institutional care to the present in an effort to aid the student in developing an appreciation for some of the current challenges that exist. Some of the lessons to be learned from history, which could be transferred to other clinical settings, are outlined.

Characteristics of long-term care facility residents are described. The advocacy role of the gerontological nurse in assisting residents and their families in selecting and adjusting to nursing facilities is discussed. Specific factors to consider in advocating for residents and families are offered in Display 32-1, which outlines factors to consider when selecting a nursing facility, and Display 32-2, which describes measures to help families with nursing facility admission of a relative.

The various nursing responsibilities within long-term care facilities are discussed. Rather than portrayed as overwhelming, these responsibilities are presented as opportunities for gerontological nurses to influence care in a variety of roles.

A new paradigm for long-term care is introduced that promotes a holistic healing-focused model rather than the current biomedical one. Figure 32-1 demonstrates a new way of looking at residents' needs. The student is challenged to reclaim nursing's healing role and create a new vision for long-term care.

■ Significant Displays, Figures, and Tables

STUDENT OBJECTIVES

After reading this chapter, the student should be able to:

1. Describe the development of long-term institutional care.

2. Discuss the problems resulting from the lack of a unique model for long-term care.

3. Identify major categories of standards described in regulations.

4. List various roles of nursing in long-term care facilities.

5. Describe hygiene, holism, and healing needs of facility residents.

■ Classroom Teaching-Learning Activities

1. Visit a long-term care facility and instruct the students to:
   - review the records of several residents and identify the types of medical and nursing diagnoses they have
   - interview at least one resident to learn about life in a facility
   - interview a family member of a resident to learn about the challenges of having a loved one in a facility
   - meet with several nursing staff to learn about the joys and frustrations of working in this setting.

2. Review a Minimum Data Set (MDS) tool and ask the students to discuss the limitations of this tool for comprehensive resident assessment.

■ Guidelines for Evaluating Critical Thinking Exercises

1.
   - dreaded form of care seen as last resort; misconception that care is custodial in nature rather than rehabilitative; miconception that families abandon loved ones who are residents of long-term care facilities; misconception that employees in nursing homes are abusive, uncaring, incompetent; media tend to highlight negative facilities
   - nurses may have misconceptions that nursing home care requires less skill and competency than nursing in other settings; nurses may not want to be affiliated with care setting that has poor image

2.
  - educate public about realities of long-term care
  - become politically active to affect change in long-term care facilities
  - achieve positions of power in long-term care sector to be able to influence change
  - define and advocate for improved quality of care and better staffing and resources

■ Test Questions

1. True or false: Early models for institutional care were developed in the United States and later replicated in European countries.
   a. true
   b. false

2. All of the following are characteristics of "total institutions"except:
   a. all individuals treated in the same manner
   b. activities conducted in different ways at different times
   c. numerous, heavily enforced rules
   d. activities focusing more on serving the needs of the institution than the needs of the individual

3. The first major government funds to aid in the construction of nursing homes was provided by the:
   a. Social Security Act
   b. Hill-Burton Act
   c. Medicare
   d. Omnibus Budget Reconciliation Act

4. True or false: It is the level of function, not the medical diagnosis, that influences the need for long-term care.
   a. true
   b. false

5. The most significant factor responsible for the growth of nursing homes between the 1960s and 1980s was:
   a. growth of the older population
   b. consumer pressure for long-term care
   c. reduction in family caregiving
   d. government reimbursement

6. True or false: The physical environment can be used as a therapeutic tool.

   a. **true**

   b. false

7. The Minimum Data Set refers to:

   a. minimum staffing levels required for a facility

   b. basic goals that must be part of every long-term care facility resident's care plan

   c. **the standardized assessment tool used for long-term care facility residents**

   d. mandatory documentation requirements for long-term care facilities

8. A characteristic of holism is:

   a. **harmony of body, mind, and spirit**

   b. cure

   c. use of alternative therapies

   d. focus on self

9. True or false: Government regulations describe the minimum standards that a facility must meet to comply with the law.

   a. **true**

   b. false

10. In the hierarchy of nursing facility residents' needs, assisting a resident to achieve deeper spiritual awareness and growth would be an action within which level of need?

    a. hygiene

    b. holism

    c. complementary

    d. **healing**

CHAPTER 33

Family Caregiving

Chapter 33 addresses the growing occurrence of family caregiving. Students are guided to dispel the myth that families forget and neglect their elder relatives and instead recognize that families are providing more direct care for longer periods of time than ever before in history.

Various family compositions are discussed. With the increased number of family structures outside the traditional nuclear family, nurses must be prepared for the diversity that exists among family units.

Family roles and relationships are described to enable the student to understand the different reactions and patterns of family dynamics that may be experienced.

In the discussion of family caregiving, the needs of the patient and the family are reviewed, with emphasis on developing a caregiving plan that serves the best interests of all. Display 33-2 lists suggestions for nurses to aid family caregivers.

Elder abuse is discussed as it relates to caregiving stress. Ways in which abuse can be manifested are listed.

Rather than just highlight the problems of family caregiving, the chapter also points to the fact that caregiving can be a positive experience.

■ Significant Displays, Tables, and Figures

Types of Assistance Provided by Families to Their Elder Members (Display 33-1)
Nursing Strategies to Assist Family Caregivers (Display 33-2)
Nursing Diagnosis Highlight: Altered Family Processes

STUDENT OBJECTIVES

After reading this chapter, the student should be able to:

1. List various family structures to which the older adult can belong.

2. Describe the roles that can be filled by family members and implications for nursing.

3. Discuss measures that can assist family caregivers in protecting the health of themselves and the patient.

4. List forms of elder abuse and actions nurses can take when they identify abuse.

▪ Classroom Teaching-Learning Activities

1. Ask the students to discuss the impact that caring for an older relative could have on their lives.

2. Identify resources in the local community for assisting families with caregiving.

3. Have the students outline their own family tree and next to the names of family members, describe the roles they assume in the family.

4. List examples of questions nurses can ask patients to learn about family composition, roles, and relationships.

▪ Guidelines for Evaluating Critical Thinking Exercises

1.
   - forfeiture of job or change in work schedule
   - modification of home to accommodate needs of elder
   - financial burden
   - added responsibilities
   - diminished leisure time, social activities

2. Discuss problems inherent in this situation and approaches that could be used. Encourage students to discuss how a similar situation would affect their own lives.

3.
   - "giving back" to person who has given to or helped them
   - living their faith in service to others
   - setting model for younger family members
   - avoiding regrets and guilt

4. Guide students in exploring resources in local community.

■ Test Questions

1. An accurate statement about the elderly and their families is:

   a. Most elders enjoy regular contact with their children.

   b. Most elders live in the same household with a child and his or her family.

   c. There is increased friction between husbands and wives in old age.

   d. As compared with previous generations, families provide less care for their elders.

2. Which of the following is not considered elder abuse?

   a. withholding medication and care

   b. intentional mismanagement of assets

   c. refusing to accept caregiving responsibilities

   d. inflicting pain

3. All of the following are acceptable strategies to assist family caregivers except:

   a. introducing care options

   b. assessing the impact of caregiving on the entire family unit

   c. guiding the family to realistically viewing the situation

   d. avoiding overwhelming them by omitting discussions of potential problems

4. List at least five different family structures that can exist.

   Unmarried couples, married couples, same-sex couples, couples with children, single parent and children, groups of unrelated individuals, siblings, multi-generations

5. True or false: Most elderly would prefer to live in the home of an adult child than alone.

   a. true

   b. false

6. True or false: Lifelong relationships are a good predictor of family relationships in late life.

   a. true

   b. false

7. True or false: Although this is rapidly changing, formal (paid) agencies provide most care to older adults, not family caregivers.

   a. true

   b. false

8. List three reasons for altered family processes.

   Illness or injury of family member, change in dependency level of family member, addition or loss of family member, relocation, reduced income, break in religious or cultural practices

9. In most situations, elder abuse is related to:

   a. a history of family violence

   b. a covert desire to place the elder in an institution

   c. psychopathology of the elder or the abuser

   d. caregiver stress

10. Explain the importance of understanding the roles various family members fill.

    Aids in understanding factors contributing to dysfunction/pathology, provides insight into family caregiving potential

CHAPTER 34

Death and Dying

Chapter 34 reviews issues pertaining to death and dying in our society. The student is aided to see the reasons for some of the difficulty people have in facing death.

The coping mechanisms that people may use as they are dying are reviewed with suggestions for nursing interventions at each stage. The way in which family, friends, and caregivers of the dying individual use these coping mechanisms also are discussed.

In addition to the physical and emotional needs of the dying person, spiritual needs are described. Table 34-2 lists basic differences among religions in beliefs and practices related to death so that the student can gain sensitivity to differences.

The chapter addresses the needs of survivors after a patient has died and the important role nurses can play in this respect. Nursing staff are among the survivors in need of support who are included in this discussion.

■ Significant Displays, Tables, and Figures

Hospice (Display 34-1)
Pain Management for the Dying Patient (Display 34-2)
Nursing Diagnoses Related to Death and Dying (Table 34-1)
Religious Beliefs and Practices Related to Death (Table 34-2)
Changes in Birth and Death Rates from 1950 to 1985 (Figure 34-1)
Example of a Pain Record (Figure 34-3)

STUDENT OBJECTIVES

After reading this chapter, the student should be able to:

1. Discuss the difficulty people have in facing death.

2. Describe the coping mechanisms people use in facing death and related nursing interventions.

3. List physical care needs of dying individuals and related nursing interventions.

4. Discuss ways in which nurses can support family and friends of dying individuals.

▪ Classroom Teaching-Learning Activities

1. Ask the students to share experiences concerning their own families' beliefs and practices regarding death.

2. Invite a hospice nurse to discuss his or her observations about the needs of dying individuals and their families.

3. List actions that nurses could advise widows or widowers to take following the death of a spouse, including agencies that must be notified, sources of support, and meal planning.

▪ Guidelines for Evaluating Critical Thinking Exercises

1.
   - death is removed from everyday life
   - most deaths occur outside of home
   - death may be viewed as failure of medical system rather than natural part of life
   - may lack belief in life after death

2. Spirituality involves relationship with higher power that transcends individual; religion involves practices related to a belief system.

3.
   - protects their rights to have their own wishes respected
   - prevents confusion, conflict, and problems for family

4.
   - grief, depression
   - anger at patient's family, facility, caregivers

▪ Test Questions

1. A dying patient is withdrawing, crying, making comments regarding the regret she will feel at not getting to see her grandchildren grow, and otherwise showing signs of depression. Your best action is to:

   a. tell her "You will soon be with God, so don't worry."

   b. encourage her to cheer up and make the most of her final days.

   c. **hold her hand and allow her to express her feelings**

   d. afford her privacy and time alone to work through these feelings

2. Regarding pain management in dying individuals, an accurate statement is:

   a. Measures should be taken to prevent pain.

   b. Pain is seldom a concern among persons near death.

   c. Physical or psychological dependency on analgesics should be avoided.

   d. Analgesics are seldom effective in dying persons.

3. One month after the death of her spouse, an older widow could be expected to:

   a. have a reawakening of interest in life

   b. experience intense grief

   c. not yet feel the impact of the death

   d. reject assistance that may be offered

4. Discuss three reasons for adults of all ages having more difficulty accepting death than have previous generations.

   • death is removed from everyday life

   • most deaths occur outside of home

   • death may be viewed as failure of medical system rather than natural part of life

   • may lack belief in life after death

5. True or false: Most deaths occur in the home, not in a hospital or other institutional setting.

   a. true

   b. false

For questions 6 to 10, state each of the stages of dying as described by Kübler-Ross and give an example of a nursing measure that can be effective for the stage.

6. Denial: accept behaviors, leave open door for honest dialogue

7. Anger: avoid reacting to anger, anticipate needs, provide safe environment for feelings to be expressed

8. Bargaining: avoid judging, protect from harmful commitments

9. Depression: be available, help family understand

10. Acceptance: provide comfort, be available, support family

Legal Aspects
of Gerontological Nursing

Chapter 35 highlights the unique legal risks of gerontological nursing practice. The types of laws that govern gerontological nursing in various practice settings are discussed. Commonly encountered issues that present legal risks and measures to reduce risks are reviewed; these issues include malpractice, consent, competency, staff supervision, drugs, restraints, telephone orders, no-code orders, advance directives, and abuse.

■ Significant Displays, Tables, and Figures

Sources of Laws (Display 35-1)
Acts That Could Result in Legal Liability for Nurses (Display 35-2)
Recommendations for Reducing the Risk of Malpractice (Display 35-3)
Types of Decision-Making Authority That Individuals Can Legally Possess Over Patients (Display 35-4)

STUDENT OBJECTIVES

After reading this chapter, the student should be able to:

1. List legal risks in gerontological nursing practice and ways to minimize them.

2. Discuss ways to protect the legal rights of older adults.

■ Classroom Teaching-Learning Activities

1. Discuss the legal risks that could arise in the following situations and measures nurses can take to reduce them:

   a. An unconscious older man is brought into the emergency department alone and is being resuscitated. His family has not been able to be reached, and it is not known if he has an advance directive. The physician is contemplating the use of life support equipment.

   b. A nursing home resident regularly wanders out of the facility into the neighboring community at all hours of the day and night. Her family does not want her restrained.

c. You are the charge nurse for the west wing of a nursing facility. Fifteen minutes into the shift, you are informed that the east wing charge nurse did not come to work and you must cover that wing in addition to your own because there will be no nurse on the unit otherwise. You believe and state that you are shorthanded on your own wing and will not be able to spend any time on the other wing. Your supervisor tells you that "you don't have to worry about actually spending time on the other unit because the nursing assistants will take care of everything."

▪ Guidelines for Evaluating Critical Thinking Exercises

1.

- older patients typically have multiple problems and are at high risk for complications
- nurses often work independently in geriatric care settings

2. Contact legal division of state agency on aging.

3. Discuss advantages to elder in assuring personal desires are known and followed.

4.

- take issue to the immediate supervisor's supervisor
- initiate elder abuse complaint
- discuss importance of not using restraints, including description of risks associated with restraint use; document topics covered in the discussion; and ask daughter to sign document acknowledging that she understands implications of her decision.

▪ Test Questions

1. All of the following conditions must be present for malpractice to be proven except:
   a. duty
   b. direct responsibility
   c. negligence
   d. injury

2. Mr. Leonard, 82 years old, is in need of surgery, and the surgeon is explaining the procedure to him and his wife. Mr. Leonard looks somewhat overwhelmed; his wife suggests that the surgeon review the procedure with their daughter, who is a nurse, and allow her to sign or refuse for Mr. Leonard. You know that the best action is for the surgeon to:
   a. obtain consent from the daughter
   b. obtain consent from the wife
   c. obtain consent from Mr. Leonard
   d. have Mr. Leonard declared incompetent and obtain consent from the guardian

3. A legally sound no-code order is:
   a. written in an advance directive
   b. developed by the health care team
   c. written in the care plan
   d. written by the physician

4. A law enacted by government legislation, such as a nurse practice act, is a
   a. regulation
   b. statute
   c. attorney general opinion
   d. court decision

5. Unlawful restraint of a patient can be an example of:
   a. false imprisonment
   b. assault
   c. battery
   d. malfeasance

6. List three reasons for the risk of legal problems being high in gerontological nursing.
   • older patients typically have multiple problems and are at high risk for complications
   • nurses often work independently in geriatric care settings
   • litigious society

7. In order to grant informed consent for a procedure, the patient should have a description of all of the following except:
   a. alternatives to the procedure
   b. description of the procedure
   c. risks
   d. other agencies/providers who perform the procedure

8. A man in an early stage of Alzheimer's disease, who is able to comprehend and make informed decisions, states that he wants to make legal arrangements for his brother to be able to make decisions on his behalf when he is no longer competent to make decisions. The type of document that could achieve this person's goal is:

   a. durable power of attorney

   b. power of attorney

   c. guardian of property

   d. guardian of person

9. True or false: The Patient Self-Determination Act required that all health care institutions had to obtain informed consent prior to doing diagnostic and treatment procedures that exceeded routine care.

   a. true

   b. false

10. True or false: Threatening to withhold care from an older adult is an example of elder abuse.

    a. true

    b. false

CHAPTER **36**

Ethics of Caring

Chapter 36 discusses changes in the profession and in society that create ethical dilemmas for nurses, including the expanded role of the nurse, new fiscal constraints, and the growing number of elderly in society.

Utilitarianism, egoism, relativism, and naturalism are presented as philosophies that influence ethical thinking. The ethical principles that guide nursing practice are discussed; these principles are beneficence, nonmaleficence, justice, fidelity, and autonomy. Dilemmas that arise in the application of these principles are reviewed. The student is given recommendations for making ethical decisions and resolving ethical dilemmas.

■ Significant Displays, Tables, and Figures

Code for Nurses (Display 36-1)
Ethical Dilemmas in Gerontological Nursing Practice (Display 36-2)

STUDENT OBJECTIVES

After reading this chapter, the student should be able to:

1. List factors that have increased ethical dilemmas for nurses.

2. Discuss various philosophies as to what is right and wrong.

3. Describe ethical principles guiding nursing practice.

4. Identify measures to assist in making ethical decisions.

■ Classroom Teaching-Learning Activities

1. Ask the students to describe issues related to the care of individual elders and the elderly as a population that could create ethical dilemmas.

2. List and discuss measures health care workers can use to resolve ethical dilemmas.

3. List and discuss the types of issues that could be referred to an ethics committee.

■ Guidelines for Evaluating Critical Thinking Exercises

1.
- family
- experience
- education
- friends
- religious beliefs

2.
- responsibility to preserve life versus respecting information shared in confidence
- duty to patient versus employer
- honoring rules/needs of organization versus contributing to potential suffering of employee
- valuing one generation's needs over the other
- ageism versus need to ration limited resources

■ Test Questions

1. Eighty-five-year-old Mrs. Jennings lives in a roach-infested house in a high-crime area of a city. The nurse discusses with Mrs. Jennings moving to a new senior apartment complex, and she flatly refuses. Despite the information the nurse shares, Mrs. Jennings insists that she has no intention of moving. The nurse tells her that as a gerontological nurse she has a better understanding of these matters, has assessed that the senior apartments would be advantageous for Mrs. Jennings, and will go ahead and enter Mrs. Jennings' name on the waiting list because the nurse "knows she'll come around to her way of thinking." The nurse's behavior is an example of:
   a. autonomy
   b. nonmaleficence
   c. beneficence
   d. paternalism

2. In the above situation, if the nurse had respected Mrs. Jennings' decision it would be an example of:
   a. autonomy
   b. nonmaleficence
   c. beneficence
   d. paternalism

3. The Code for Nurses that offers ethical guidelines for nursing practice has been developed by:

   a. federal law

   b. state boards of nursing practice

   c. the American Nurses Association

   d. the Department of Health and Human Services

4. List three reasons for new ethical dilemmas in gerontological nursing.

   Persons are living longer, health care resources are finite and being rationed, quality-of-life issues have generated open discussions of euthanasia and suicide, scarce resources are fueling intergenerational conflict

5. True or false: Most individuals view the same ethical dilemma in a similar manner.

   a. true

   b. false

6. List three factors that can help in making ethical decisions.

   Discuss with ethics committee, review code of ethics, encourage patients' expression of desires, be aware of own values

   For questions 7 to 10, match the term with the definition that best describes it from the list below:

   a. to be fair and treat people equally

   b. to respect our word and duty to our patients

   c. to do no harm

   d. to respect patients' freedoms, preferences, and rights

   e. to do good for patients

7. beneficence: e

8. justice: a

9. fidelity: b

10. autonomy: d

CHAPTER 37

The Continuum of Services

Chapter 37 introduces students to the wide range of practice settings that provide challenging opportunities for nurses to work with older adults. Rather than limit their view of gerontological nursing practice settings as being nursing homes or adult day care centers, students are encouraged to see opportunities to work with aging individuals in new settings such as parishes, group homes, and telephone reassurance programs.

Practice settings along the continuum are described with specific information about locating these services. In addition to conventional services, nontraditional services such as homeopathy and acupuncture are mentioned to increase students' awareness of consumers' growing interest in this arena of services.

Factors to consider when selecting services for elderly clients are described. The selection of services based on the individual's needs is emphasized. Students are assisted in identifying resources of benefit to clients by the listing of resources at the end of the chapter.

■ Significant Displays, Tables, and Figures

Functions of the Gerontological Nurse (Display 37-1)
Measures That Enhance the Quality of Hospital Care for the Elderly (Display 37-2)
Continuum of Care Services for Older Adults (Figure 37-2)

STUDENT OBJECTIVES

After reading this chapter, the student should be able to:

1. List major functions of the gerontological nurse.
2. Describe various practice settings for gerontological nurses.
3. Describe the continuum of services available to older adults.
4. Discuss factors that influence service selection for older adults.

■ Classroom Teaching-Learning Activities

1. Discuss the various functions of gerontological nurses and potential new practice roles in the future.

163

2. Describe the continuum of services for older adults in their local communities.

3. Discuss consumer interest in nontraditional services and nursing's role in helping consumers use these services wisely.

■ Guidelines for Evaluating Critical Thinking Exercises

1.
- most problems/needs of elders fall within realm of nursing
- nurses tend to have holistic approach

2.
- initially patient can go to nursing facility for rehabilitation, then be discharged home with home health services, and then use adult day care services
- caregiver aid resources in community can be consulted
- family may benefit from support group, counseling

3.
- search models in other community
- elicit involvement of interested individuals and groups (senior groups, churches, health departments, aging services)
- meet with local political leaders and directors of health and social service agencies

■ Test Questions

1. The fastest-growing component of community-based long-term care is:
   a. **adult day care**
   b. group homes
   c. the wellness center
   d. over-60 counseling services

2. A goal of the gerontological nurse in working with the health care team is to:
   a. direct and evaluate provision of services by all disciplines
   b. demonstrate nursing's competencies in the provision of services
   c. **collaborate in the delivery of services**
   d. gain a position of authority within the team

3. Which is not an accurate statement concerning the elderly's use of health care services?

    a. Most acute medical beds are filled by older patients.

    b. Older adults use home health services less than other age groups.

    c. About 40% of the elderly will spend some time in a nursing home.

    d. More than one-third of all surgical patients are over age 65.

4. Residential care facilities and personal care homes are examples of:

    a. assisted living

    b. nursing homes

    c. home monitoring

    d. day treatment

5. If an older client displays an interest in an alternative therapy such as acupuncture or homeopathy, the nurse should:

    a. avoid discussion or encouragement of such a therapy

    b. identify a conventional therapy that can substitute for the alternative

    c. explain that alternative therapies are ineffective and a waste of money

    d. educate the client about the risks and benefits of the therapy

6. Persons with the capacity for independent self-care would benefit best from which type of service?

    a. preventive and ancillary

    b. supportive

    c. partial and intermittent care

    d. complete and continuous care

7. An older couple tell you that they have heard about reverse annuity mortgages and believe this program could assist them in increasing their monthly income. To help the couple learn more, you would refer them to:

    a. the Social Security Administration

    b. the Veterans Administration

    c. the Department of Housing and Urban Development

    d. a banking institution

8. True or false: The American Nurses Association has taken the position that professional nurses make excellent case managers.

    a. true

    b. false

9. The Omnibus Budget Reconciliation Act of 1987 (OBRA) most profoundly reformed care in which type of setting?

   a. inpatient hospital

   b. outpatient hospital

   c. nursing home

   d. home health

10. Explain what is meant by the statement *Services should exist to allow the older adult to move along the continuum of care as needed.*

    There should be many options to address needs as elders require more or less services

CHAPTER 38

Challenges of the Future

Challenges of the Future, the final chapter of the text, stimulates the student to consider the many possibilities for future gerontological nursing opportunities. The challenges are summarized as advancing research, educating caregivers, developing new roles, balancing priorities, and promoting creative holistic practices. Nurses are encouraged to assume leadership in the continued development of the specialty.

■ Student Objectives

After reading this chapter, the student should be able to:

1. Describe ways in which nurses can encourage and support gerontological nursing research.

2. List practical opportunities for educating caregivers.

3. Identify possible new roles for gerontological nurses.

4. Discuss ways in which gerontological nurses can assist with cost containment while protecting the rights of the elderly.

5. Describe the significance of holistic practices to nursing the elderly.

■ Classroom Teaching-Learning Exercises

1. Identify various agencies that provide services (e.g., health, housing, social) for older adults and discuss existing and potential nursing roles in these agencies.

2. Ask the students to develop job descriptions for the following roles:

   a. wellness clinic nurse in a senior apartment complex

   b. chronic care case manager in private practice

   c. aging educator in elementary through secondary school systems

■ Guidelines for Evaluating Critical Thinking Exercises

1. Guide students in locating local chapters of the National Gerontological Nursing Association, the National Association of Directors of Nursing in Long-Term Care, and other gerontological-focused groups.

2. Have students brainstorm on possible areas for research.

3.
   - empowers consumers and increases responsibility for self-care
   - less expense, natural treatments may be used
   - preventive care is emphasized

4. Have students brainstorm on the variety of functions that could be demonstrated in these various roles.

■ Test Questions

1. When looking for new roles, gerontological nurses show leadership by:
   a. following the lead of new roles in medicine
   b. looking at needs and developing roles accordingly
   c. practicing within the confines of traditional roles and settings
   d. asking administrators to create new roles for them

2. The hospital is looking for ways to reduce costs. The least helpful response of the hospital nurse to this measure is to:
   a. participate in cost review and evaluation measures
   b. explore ways to reduce costs
   c. test innovative staffing practices
   d. threaten to strike if the nursing budget is affected

3. Describe three factors that caused gerontological nurses to have low status and power in the past.
   - emphasis on acute care through educational process
   - gerontological nursing associated with nursing homes and stigma associated with nursing home care
   - gerontological nursing was not taught in nursing schools
   - gerontological nursing a relatively new specialty as compared with other nursing specialties

4. Describe one way in which the gerontological nurse can advance research in the specialty without conducting it herself or himself.

   Communicate results of concern and potential research topics to nurse researchers, support research efforts, keep abreast of and implement research findings

5. List three new roles that gerontological nurses could develop.

   Preretirement couselor, chronic care case manager, aging educator for gyms, etc.

6. Describe three opportunities to provide education to advance gerontological caregiving knowledge.

   Guest lectures in schools and community, writing articles, leading support group, initiating network for caregivers, etc.

For questions 7 to 10, state and describe four subspecialties of gerontological nursing.

   Geropsychiatry, geriatric rehabilitation, geriatric surgery, nursing administration in long-term care, adult day services, etc.